# A New Weigh
# In 21 Days

*Transform Your
Image
Transform Your
Life*

# CONTENTS

# INTRODUCTION

"How'd we get so fat?" A beautiful woman casually asked me this question as we sat in plush seats in an elegant theater waiting for the evening's concert to begin. Her question summed up a chatty exchange that we were having to entertain ourselves until show time. Our conversation had begun with positive comments about what other folks were wearing and moved rather naturally to the subject and popularity of cosmetic surgery, makeovers, and then we went there! "There" is today's hottest topic, our national weight epidemic. So back to the question again, "How'd we get so fat?" A dead silence was all that filled the empty space now.

The curtain rolled up; it was show time, but for me, it was her question that was playing, like a monotonous melody in my head: "How'd we get so fat?" Finally, the answer to that question resounded loudly in my head. We have attracted weight into our society and we weren't even aware of our invitation to bulge. You might say, no, how is that possible? There were no signs along the way, no desire to be weighted.

Yes, our attention to obesity in the beginning was unconscious, but grew to be consistent and obsessive. We strongly supported the idea of obesity by eating fat, talking fat, acting fat, seeing ourselves as fat and yes, here we are fulfilling our beliefs and living out our newly perceived, transformed lifestyles; we as a country are overweight/fat. There it is, the magnetic attraction of thought, our mass mental attraction to weight.

It began about forty-some years ago. We as Americans started talking about and focusing our attention on obesity. Do you remember Twiggy, the real-life wafer-thin model from England? The only thing big about her were her eyes. She looked like a poster child promoting "skinny" as the new "in" thing. But never mind, in the '60s, we wanted "that" look.

We are demonstrating obesity on a national level! Everywhere we look we experience the latest fad diets, books, spas, clinics, on magazine covers, TV shows—even celebrities have formally joined the ranks of dieters. Our careers, social life, even our personal relationships are affected by obesity. Most importantly, our health is dangerously subject to obesity. Heart problems, diabetes, stroke, arthritis, are only a few of the many serious health conditions caused by or exacerbated by fat. Folks are wiring their teeth, subjecting themselves to major surgery and literally dying for the look.

Interest in weight represents a cross-section of every age group, all cultures and ethnic groups in our country. Billions of dollars are spent each year on weight and yet 71% of us think we are overweight and 67% of us are, not counting the 17% of our kids who are now obese. Because of this, our life expectancy rates are droping.

Fashion market geniuses have swooped down, like eagles, considering the American culture as fat prey. They have sold the concept that everyone can have "IT": the right look. The acceptable IQ of the masses has been raised to an incredible all-time high. By the way, the new definition of IQ is image quotient, you know, the way one's image measures up. Up to what, who, why? The diet corporations have become the authority on image; they dictate how we in America "should"—oh, no, *must* look! No fat trimmed here.

These weight marketing gurus have become to image what Bill Gates was to personal computers. They sold the idea that you gotta have one… the slim body. The masses bought into it, and still continue to focus on weight and all that goes with it. We have created a "fat" nation, a national epidemic, second only to cigarette smoking as a preventable disease.

Most of us would agree: it's not how we got so fat but how we get fat-free. Free of the burdens, the challenges and yes, the health threats caused by fat. There was that question glaring at me still. How do we become "fat-free"? Those who are fat free fall into only 5% of those who attempt to change their weight. When asked how they do it, their answers are always based upon the total image formula; Transform Your Image, (change what you think, see and believe is your truth about your image), Transform Your Life (demonstrate/ live that new belief).

Hmmm, they had transformed their inner lives, their outer experiences and had expressed a new confidence, a new sense of value. Yes, the answer: "Transform Your Image, Transform Your Life."

You are invited to participate in an experience that transforms your image, your weight and yes, your life. Weight will change when you change your total approach to it and lifestyle as a result of it. You may say, "Sure, easy for you to say." Yes, the question of how we become fat-free is a question asked by millions of people across the country. Here's your solution.

# Transform Your Image, Transform Your Life

Would you participate in an experience, a program that transforms your life, your health and weight permanently in just 21 days? Do you want to get over weight—yes, that's right, over it? Over the emotional weight, the mental weight as well as the physical weight. Your life will change when you change it. You are invited to discover that change or transformation related to weight is the direct result of the way you think, listen to those thoughts and follow them into positive action. You can change the way you think…it happens from the inside out. Oh we are busy working to change the effects of our lives. But ironically, when we look at the effects we have created rather than the causes behind the effects, we support the effects and keep them alive. What you put your attention on is what you must experience. So in this 21-day practice, we put our attention on the solutions and the desired success. Our actions support the solutions. So, we experience success in transforming our image, and yes, the weight as well.

What are the effects of our lives? They are the physical results of what we believe, perceive as real, or see as truth. These physical results are the body, the environment, people in our lives, emotions, challenges/conditions and habits. Many of us feel we are victims of these effects/results. We sometimes believe that we are stuck in our habits.

Of all the habits to get over, weight is the most challenging and the most rewarding. No other habit is so directly related to life. If you are an alcoholic, you can avoid alcohol. You don't need it to live. The same is true for smoking, drugs, and other compulsive habits. Even though these habits may be connected to the body and its emotions, and are very difficult to give up or modify, you CAN give them up and still live. You cannot give up eating and live. So you must face all day long what you feel is the very obstacle that blocks your path to success: food. Yes, food seems like the enemy, the enemy that you must deal with every day. A comedian once said, "Ya know, I am in love with the one that I hate." You are not alone. The masses are struggling with weight issues.

People are, for the most part, bound by their outer experiences and think that what they see on the outside is who they are. They may feel that they are locked into that life, that experience. You are not just your body, your emotions or your thoughts. You are the sum of all of these parts of you plus an inner life as well. Are you aware of your inner life? This inner life is who you really are. This "who" gives you guidance, direction and support. It can direct/guide you to the creation of a new life style, a new image and a new weight.

We have all experienced hearing a voice in our heads, thoughts, a hunch, an intuition (guide).These experiences are your connection to your inner life, a central Self. Your inner Self is referred to as "The Boss" in this 21-day experience. Your personality, the ego can make choices based upon this guidance, "The Boss". Through these personal choices you create physical results You don't need a popular diet, or an expert to tell you what is best for you relating to your weight, image or life style. You have an internal guide that knows what is best for you, it's built in. When you listen, it suggests the right foods, the right schedule that is just for Y.O.U., an acronym that spells our...Your Own Uniqueness. You willl learn to listen to "The Boss" to create a new lifestyle that is not only best for you but unique to you. "The Boss" will help you to get over weight, experience a new weigh..

.The system is a 21-day experience. It is a day-by-day practice designed to support your release of weight. You will experience a new way of life that is just right for you. You will learn about your belief systems, and discover your unique patterns, and how they shape your life. In this short period of 21 days, you will learn and practice mental concepts that can remove old patterns about you that may have placed blocks and barriers in the way of your personal success.

You need not be concerned about image or weight. Getting over it is an inside action that begins with you believing in and loving yourself as you are. You are encouraged to be inner directed. You can live a life of freedom, free to be "over" weight forever. Yes, over it, let it go! Experience the perfect self that is in charge of your life, the self that is "over" weight for now and always. Congratulations, you are "The Boss"; stay the course, Transform Your Image, Transform Your Life, experience a New Weigh in 21 days.

# Instructions

Before beginning this new lifestyle, take a look at your present routines, your eating habits, your health and your emotional states. Your success in this experience depends upon the states of these areas of your life. This is not a quick fix or one-shot program. Many times you desire a change in your life but are not prepared physically, mentally or emotionally to follow through with what it takes to be successful. Your current lifestyle, environment, schedule, food, resources and physical ability need to be considered. You can clear away all of the obstacles that have sabotaged your success in other endeavors.

You will experience success day by day, one day at a time. It is a very present-centered practice, a new way of living that deserves your full attention and discipline, one moment at a time. Anything will work if you work it, you know, do the exercises, read the material and practice, practice. Your success in any program will take commitment, responsibility and love. Only you can move the blocks and old patterns in your life and change the flow of your lifestyle. You must be willing to go beyond what you think is real to a new truth, a new pattern. Yes, by manipulating the interferences and blocks that are in your way, you can redirect the flow of your life, you can create your freedom. The change is yours to make. You can choose what you see as your reality. The outcome: *your* best health and image; a new weigh.

. This is a 21-day experience designed to be your formula for success. It is a positive makeover, a natural and permanent new image created by you for you. The lifestyles related to image are the most challenging and yes, the most rewarding when managed. No other lifestyle is so directly connected to health, esteem, confidence and personal success. Now is the time to break the diet cycle. It happens through three major concepts that are presented throughout the book.

## *Transform Your Mind*

Identify and use your inner image—your thoughts, attitudes and beliefs—this is a critical component. However, it must be balanced by action, a conscious and deliberate change in the outer activities as well. You establish a total image, the one that is ideal for you. This happens on the inside first as a belief about yourself is validated by your follow through and care for your body, appearance and environment. The final touch: a new attitude, body and image...

## *Transform Your Body, Your Health*

A new life, a new you begin with your health. You are being introduced to an all-natural, 21$^{st}$ century lifestyle that transforms your body through; your thinking, eating and natural exercise .This is a 21-day practice of easy nutritious menu options. You will learn about body types, body rhythms, how they affect your eating styles and how to create your very own personal eating system. You will learn to listen to "The Boss." There will be a feeling of exhilaration and inspiration about the 10 to 20 pounds released during this easy 21 day solution. Got your attention?

## *Transform Your Spirit*

Your total image is very critical to your transformation. Your personal wardrobe, skin care, make up and carriage are contributors to your own unique presentation and will be part of the total image practice. You will look as good as you feel. and experience high energy, high esteem. You will look like you love yourself every time you step out. This feeling is cause to your personal success.

It is time to give up the miracle diets and the get-thin-quick schemes, the untested and the untrue. Now is the time for transformation in your life. An honest system based on good things like personal focus, smart choices and feeling great about yourself... Here you have a formula for success that supports your resolve to see the plan through, one that helps you to take charge, get results. Challenge yourself to do things differently. You will experience weight release and a new image, a new weigh. Are you ready for a permanent makeover? This is your opportunity to make it happen

Here's how:

## Components

Each day consists of the following components:

### Part I:  Transform Your Image

The mental image component presents practical information, ideas and concepts that are designed to build your personal resources and arm you with the tools needed to change your mind, emotions, attitudes and beliefs about weight and image. There are exercises designed to transform your thinking. You will practice behavior skills that move you from limiting habits and defeating attitudes, to positive approaches to weight management and self-acceptance.

## Part II:  The Physical Image

### The Body/Health and Image

In this section you will focus on nutrition and menu ideas.  You will also be introduced to resources, and concepts of body types, body rhythm, personal carriage, skin care, and self-presentation.  You will learn about healthy eating, handling special events and personal environments that contribute to physical health and well-being.

### Recommendations

Before beginning any weight-changing program it is recommended that you inform your health-care provider and schedule a physical exam.

### Listen to the Boss:

You will learn to listen to the "Boss."  We all have an internal life that guides and directs our actions. This inner life has been defined as intuition, a hunch, self-talk, a guide and many other names.  We will be referring to it as the "Boss." This internal Boss, like an external one, can guide, supervise, direct, and reward you.  Because it's so personal, your own Boss can direct you to what's best for you, when it's best, and can lovingly support your decisions.  It's personal and particular to you and your needs.  Learning to listen to the Boss takes practice. You may be like one of the participants who said, "I just don't hear things in my head. It sounded spooky to me".  Then one day, I was driving down the street when I had a hunch, a feeling that I was going the wrong way.  I followed my mind and turned around.  Then it hit me.  Oh...this is what the book means by the Boss.  So I began to be aware of my hunches and followed them for everything. Listen to the Boss?  I can do that, I did it, and was successful in gaining health, losing weight and feeling good about myself. This activity is the foundation for your own unique behavior modification, "your style."  It is designed for and by you. Because of this you will succeed.

## Part III:  Transform Your Life

The total image represents an integration of all of the parts of your life.  You are successful when you change all areas of your life, your mental, physical and spiritual (unique source/energy, higher power).  The total image is your "essence."  It is fashion, style, skin care, communication, you as your best self, expressing, being it.

## Just For You (Y.O.U.)

Each day there is an activity or exercise that is just for you.  This "you," spelled out is an acronym, Y your, O own U uniqueness.  This exercise is a special gift to you.  Do something for yourself every day for 21 days and watch your self-esteem and confidence soar!  Remember, you are important, you are special, you are loved by the most important person in your life, you!

### *Menu Options*
*Contributed by Susan Hoag-Stophel Licensed Nutritionist*

In this 21-day experience, you are encouraged to listen to the "Boss" (your internal guide) to select foods, physical exercise and behavior that transform your weight.  In order to support your healthy eating practice, 21 days of menu options are included.  You may choose to use these menus or follow your own.  Be sure to plan your menus and shop your plan before each week.  Having a plan supports your resolve to stick to healthy eating.  You choose!

These meals and snacks are safe for everyone in good health.  However, no one should undertake any weight-loss program without consulting with his or her physician.

These meals and snacks are presented as menu options each day.  The menus are nutritionally balanced, high in fiber and nutrients, calorie counted, and low in salt and sugar.  They contain carbohydrates that are low on the glycemic index, which means these carbohydrates burn and are used efficiently in the human body and keep physiological hunger away.  This program is high in protein and low in fat and cholesterol.

You can repeat a day that contains the meals and snacks that you like.  Make it easy.  Find your favorites.  Enjoy!  It is important to:

1. Portion and time your meals and snacks so there is no more than a four-hour time gap between meals.

   *Portioning and timing forces your body to burn instead of store.*

2. Use no-salt seasoning suggestions instead of salt: Mrs. Dash seasonings, Parsley Patch seasonings, Lifehouse seasonings, granulated garlic, powdered onion, rice vinegar, lemon, tumeric, curry, cumin, Tabasco sauce, oregano, paprika, black pepper, white pepper.

3. Prepare your shopping list. You are preplanning for success.

   *Plan an ample inventory for home, work, and your car.*

4. Vitamins: Make sure you take a multivitamin, calcium and magnesium each day to ensure optimum nutrition. *Check with your physician for proper dosage.*

## Recommendations

Before beginning any weight-changing program it is recommended that you inform your health-care provider and schedule a physical exam.There is no perfect way to achieve success using these menus. Everything that you do makes a positive difference!

## Exercises

The value of movement cannot be measured. Our bodies are regulated and maintained by motion. Every cell and atom in your body rotates and moves in cycles. If you are not active, you slow down the natural movement of your body. This sluggish system causes major problems in circulation, respiration, water retention, digestion and elimination. Your health depends upon these systems functioning at full energy.

We must then set up a daily routine for movement/exercise. Whatever physical condition you are in won't stop your participation. You can do some form of exercise. If you already have an exercise routine, continue with it. If you do not have a plan, use the 21 days of simple exercises that are included. If these don't work, ask your health-care provider for suggestions. Do the exercises daily for optimum results.

## Insights and Action

You are invited to write out your insight for the day (as you would a journal entry). There is a form included at the end of each day for this entry. An insight is what you have learned, experienced, overcome or accomplished as a result of your participation in this educational experience. What idea, "ah, ha," or "wow" did you receive? Write it in two or three sentences. What action did you take or what activity will you undertake as a result of that insight? Your insight and action help you to record your progress and keep track of your success in a very simple, painless way. It can also assist you in making changes in your approach to the experience as you go, rather than continuing to practice something that is not working. IF ever you doubt that you are making progress refer to your insight and action sections.

## Affirmations

It is helpful to reinforce the concepts that you have learned for the day. You are given affirmations that sum up the concept in a capsule statement that can be repeated throughout the day, in your head, heart or from your lips. Affirmations speak to your mind and build credibility, belief and ownership.

# Week One
# Commitment

Take pride in your new found power. Know that it is your energy, not force, that works for you. This energy will keep you on track and support your resolve to stick to this lifestyle for seven days. You will practice letting go of your burden of guilt, fear and anxiety about weight. You will learn to live in a simpler way, by acting from your centered self. Commit your life to a new direction, with serenity and without regrets. Invest in yourself and find your treasures right where they are, where they have always been; inside you. Remember the old adage "what you are looking for you are looking with." In this week you will take action, accept commitment and experience a new you.

| | |
|---|---|
| Day 1 | Your Inner Image |
| Day 2 | Be Inner Directed |
| Day 3 | You Are What You Think |
| Day 4 | Image Myths |
| Day 5 | One Day At Time |
| Day 6 | Get In Touch With Yourself |
| Day 7 | Action Does It |

# Day 1

**Part I:**        **Your Inner Image**

**Part II:**      **Do Not Play The Weighting Game**

**Part III:**     **Transformation Model**

## Just For You (<u>Y</u>our <u>O</u>wn Uniqueness)

Write a love letter to yourself. Mail it and open it at the end of the 21-day experience. You will be surprised at your progress.

# Day 1
## Part I:                        Your Inner Image

Most people react or respond to life from the outside in. We reach outside ourselves to find the answer to life's challenges. We seek recognition, approval and acceptance from others. Most of us compete with, compare and judge ourselves by standards, values and realities created by a few who dictate to the world that which is good, that which is right, and that which is acceptable.

How can this be when we are each unique, special individuals with built in intelligence that creates successful life experiences for each of us on a personal level? This action of directed personal success happens from the inside out.

The concept of this 21-day experience is to recognize that you have an inner life that creates, manages and maintains the perfect balance, the perfect life. This inner life regulates and creates any results that you desire in your life. Further, the concept suggests that you use words, images, visions and experiences to bring about a change in your life and that this change can be manifested permanently in 21 days. Why 21 days? Therapists, psychologists and other authorities report that new life patterns can be created in 21 days.

Identifying and using this inner image is an integral component of this program. However, it must be balanced by action, a conscious and deliberate change in the outer activities as well. You establish the total image, the one that is ideal for you.

This happens on the inside first as a belief about yourself, is validated by your follow through and care for body appearance and environment and the final touch, a new attitude and presentation.

Have you heard someone say, "Just change your ways"? How is this accomplished? Change occurs when your inner image changes or when your belief about an activity changes. In this experience you learn about the characteristics of the inner image and the use of the centered self. You will also be presented with a transformation model that will assist you in the change of your image, a model that works to get over weight.

# Day 1
## Part II:          Don't Play The Weighting Game

In recent years the concept of weighing has gone to completely obsessive behavior, for the most part. Weighing was meant to measure the state of your health. It was not meant to measure beauty or whether you have been a good or bad person. If you do not fit the old insurance figures for weight, you are made to feel guilty, as if you have failed yourself and others in some way. You do all that you can to get to that illusive, ideal weight. You play the weighting game by starving, weighing, eating, weighing, and weighing again and again, sometimes seeking approval from the scale.

At last, you can stop that cycle. When you are eating healthy, drinking at least eight glasses of water per day, cleansing the body, giving it the absolute best nutrition, breathing deeply, exercising and using affirmative attitudes, you will be the perfect body for you. You do not have to weight to be happy or weight to wear beautiful clothes. Now is the time. Don't play the weighting game.

There are seven easy ideas that can break that pattern. Get over the weighting game once and for all by following these ideas:

Sit down and eat, at a table. Make it a pleasant activity by using pretty plates, service ware, table arrangements, flowers or color. The ambiance and presentation create a pleasant experience. You are worth it!

Avoid distractions: Do not eat and watch T.V. or do other distracting activities. Put your attention on the food and the company at the table, if eating with someone.

Allow approximately three to four hours between meals, unless fasting, only fast under professional supervision. Keep your life rhythm. Do not practice eating meals after 8:00 p.m. unless it a special occasion.

Chew food thoroughly. Savor food, identify flavors and enjoy your food. If all foods are disguised with spices that are used over and over, they all begin to taste the same way. When foods do not taste the same our bodies feel something is wrong. We become accustomed to a "usual" taste, a sort of taste habit. Do not eat and drink at the same time. You may want to drink your water before your meal. It clears the passage way and is filling.

Eat two handfuls of food (your hand size). Because of bad habits, your capacity to eat incnreases, making you think that you need more to eat. The size of your stomach is about the size of your hand. Learn to eat less, you don't need to over eat. If you still feel hungry, wait for twenty minutes have a healthy snack or beverage.

Eat half of whatever it is that you want to eat and you will be half your.size. You are cutting back, but in your mind you are satisfied.

Stop eating when you are no longer hungry. Identify how it feels to be satisfied, not full. Listen to the Boss!


# Day 1
# Part III:        Transformation Model

You have learned through your parents, friends and the media that change is difficult. Some even think that change is impossible. The irony is that you are changing constantly, every moment of every day. You may ask yourself, even though I seem to be working on change, I seem to be the same, act the same and look the same. As has been stated, the outer effects of your life are what you put your attention on. You tend to think the same, act the same and, because you believe the results you see to be your reality, your belief produces the same life, the same old you. How do you break this cycle of sameness or what seems like a "rut"? There are three methods that you use to cope with life. You can conform, reform or transform.

### Conform

To conform means to go along with your life circumstances. Let's break down the meaning of this method of coping with your life. Dr. Wayne Dyer, in his book, *You'll See It When You Believe It*, says that the root word in these three methods is "form." Form describes the physical. It represents your body, weight, bones, cells and/or any part of your physiology. The prefix con means to go along with. So, to conform can mean that you accept your body, weight, even though you may desire a change. It may be passive, subjective or defeating. It may mean you feel you are just going along. Sometimes this method is unconscious. You may be experiencing a hopeless feeling because of past failure. Conforming may also be a positive choice to accept who you are, the way you are

## Reform

Reform is what the masses of people do when a change is desired. Again "form" is the external, appearance, the physical. The prefix in this method is re, to do again, back up, repeat. When you use the reform method, you rearrange your styles (lifestyle); make your life different, most of the time temporarily. Like rearranging furniture in a room, you move things around but everything is basically the same. You reform your eating ritual (diet), you exercise, and you keep the same core thoughts, ideas and desires. You act the same, you look the same, and you are the same. Are you on a diet yo-yo, conscious at times, unconscious at other times? You know what to do, but using the same old methods creates the same old results.

## Transform

What you need to do to make a marked difference in your life is to transform. Again, look at the core of the word "form." Form is the body, it is the shape, and it is the physical structure. The prefix in this method is trans. Trans means to go beyond, or, in literal terms, "over." Place the prefix in front of "form" and the method is to go beyond form or body. Get over weight, the physical structure. Add the suffix "ation," which means "action" or result. The word transformation is a dynamic concept which means you experience the result through the action of going beyond your form. Go beyond the physical that you see to an image of your perfect body, the one that is perfect for you. See, the real you is 99 (ninety-nine) percent invisible, it is beyond form. You create your body every moment through your thoughts, vision and beliefs. How can you go about practicing the method of transformation?

*Model*          *Transform Your Image*

You must first of all be conscious (aware) that you are transformed, know that you have the ability, the responsibility (ability to respond), to see beyond the physical, the form. You have the capacity to experience what you create in your life. You must move away from desire, hope, and try, as these are words and attitudes that support your current behavior and your "stuck place." If you say, "I desire, I hope, I will try," then you are saying to yourself, "I believe I have the problem," or you would not be hoping, trying to change. You will continue to experience what you believe to be true, what you believe to be your problem. What you put your attention on is what you experience.

16

Think of the juice of a tart lemon squirting in your mouth, your mouth waters. Where is the lemon? In this case, the lemon is in your mind as an old patterned belief. When you are willing to focus beyond the obvious, then you are ready to experience other possibilities. Look at the images below. What do you see?

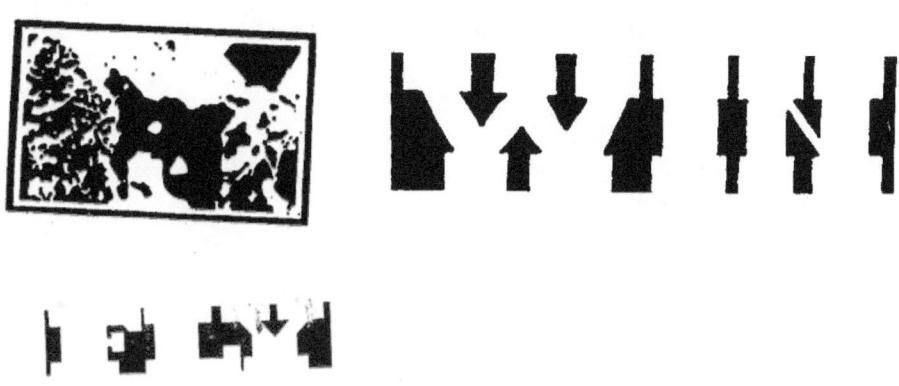

You will not be able to experience these concepts until you can focus on them, see them beyond their distorted presentations. When you do see the image, the concept becomes your new "found image". The images are WIN, FLY and a popular person. Are these images really there? Yes, they are. Is there something wrong with your perception? No, you are seeing, or not seeing, what you "believe" to be there. Can you experience these images if you try hard, if you are good, if you just want to? No, will or force does not help you to see the images. In fact, it delays the process. You are positioning yourself to transform, (go beyond) the images that you think that you see to the images that were there all of the time. When you can see (image as real) WIN, FLY and the popular person you can experience them. It is that simple. What you see and believe as your reality becomes your experience. You will and must experience it. In fact, once you experience the image as real you cannot go back to the old image. Like the butterfly, after it has had its transformation, can never be a caterpillar again.

Create a picture in your mind of your ideal self.Each day practice seeing or imagining this ideal self along with practicing the daily exercises and activities. You need to give it time, get a mental picture or physical picture of how you want to look. Do not ask for opinions, ideas or suggestions from others. When you have the picture, write it down, or draw it, take a picture. Get a symbol of it or do whatever it takes to remind you of the ideal image of yourself daily. See it as often during the day as you can. Be patient it may take time to create the picture of your ideal self.

*Exercise:* (Indoors for 30 Minutes)
Dance to your favorites: Play your favorite tunes and *dance like no one's watching* for 30 minutes.

Insight

Action

*Affirmation:*

My body is within my mind. It is a shadow of the truth of who I really am. I created it out of my thoughts, my beliefs. I can change it through my thoughts, my beliefs.

# Menu Options
## "Fuel for the Day"

---

**BREAKFAST**
1 cup Special K cereal (not strawberry)
2 teaspoons 100% all fruit jam
1 tablespoon sliced unsalted almonds½ banana
½ cup skim or low-fat milk

---

*Put all ingredients in a bowl*

**Snack Boost** *(in a Zip-loc snack bag)*
2 dried apricots
3 unsalted almonds

---

**LUNCH**
Tuna Sandwich:
3 oz. tuna (water packed)
1 tablespoon fat-free mayonnaise
Lettuce and tomato
2 slices of whole wheat bread

---

*Mix mayonnaise and tuna together and spread on whole-wheat bread. Place lettuce and tomato on top. Enjoy a fruit on the side.*

**Snack**
Strawberry Soy Shake:
½ cup West soy Lite soy milk (vanilla, chocolate or strawberry)
1 cup frozen or fresh strawberries
*Mix in blender until tall and frothy*

---

**DINNER**
Mexican Stuffed Potato:
1 potato (cooked until soft in microwave)
½ cup Rosarita fat-free refried beans
2 ounces cooked ground turkey
1 tablespoon low-fat shredded cheddar cheese

---

*Cook potato in microwave until it is soft. Fill potato with beans, turkey and cheese. Heat again. Salad or fruit or vegetable on the side.*

**Snack**
Grape Cheesy Fruity Muffin:
1 whole-wheat English muffin topped with
1 teaspoon Philadelphia Light cream cheese
2 teaspoons Simply Fruit jam
Grapes

**Your day was:** Approximately 1,250 calories, 2128 mg. sodium, 76 mg. cholesterol26% protein57% carbohydrates 17% fat

# Day 2

**Part I:**        **Be Inner Directed**

**Part II:**       **Get Into The Rhythm**

**Part III:**      **Be Conscious of Who You Are, Experience the "Ah, Ha."**

## Just For You (<u>Y</u>our <u>O</u>wn <u>U</u>niqueness)

Watch the movie *Trading Places*. Note the part that their believing creates for the characters. What they believed to be their lifestyles, who they are, changed their lives. When the rich man is thrown into poverty, he acts poor, believes he is, and assumes his bondage. When the poor man is given wealth, he succeeds because he *believes* he is wealthy and in charge. Other movie suggestions: *Me, Myself and Irene*, or *Cybil*.

# Day 2
## Part I.          Be Inner Directed

A repeated theme of this 21-day experience is the practice and use of your inner life, called the "I" or, lovingly, the "Boss." Your life can be managed by listening to and responding from your inner life, the "Boss". The inner "I" creates and governs the body, health, emotions and life styles through your beliefs. The outcomes or external experiences of your life are also created by these beliefs. What you see as true to you in the inner is what you must experience in your outer life. You are using this inner life whether you know it or not, but by managing it consciously you will transform it. Just as a car may be driven by an unskilled driver, ordinary driver, or a specially trained professional driver; so too, your life may be lived unconsciously with no direction, consciously by living on purpose, or with intention by practicing the art of listening to and following your inner "I" the "Boss". You can be inner directed and your body and life will reflect this transformation.

Your life is created as a direct result of what you believe and your action upon those beliefs. Scientific facts give evidence that the body, the emotions and intellect are instruments of experience. These are outcomes of your beliefs. The body, emotions and intellect are what you see, what you use, they are changeable, not "who" you are. These instruments can be dominated, disciplined or deliberately changed by the inner "I" the "Boss" "I" is simple, <u>un</u>changeable, constant and self-conscious (knows itself)

The idea that belief can transform the body is demonstrated vividly in the cases of multiple personality. When one is suffering from this disease and believes he is the "present" personality he becomes that personality completely. The body functions, structure and personality change to accommodate the belief. If, for instance the ill person is a diabetic in one personality and moves to another who isn't, the blood sugar in the body changes. The ill person can be a personality with cancer, and in the same body, with a different personality, free of cancer. The patient can be a man or woman, old or young and so on, in the same body. The changes are physical, emotional and intellectual. All because the patient <u>believes </u>he or she is that person. In the mentally healthy person the changes are subtle because you know that you are a constant identity with your body, emotions and thoughts. You say, "Well, that's just me, the way I am." You assume because you see yourself as that body or you look a certain way that it is just the way you are. The brain is a physical instrument, the thought is a creative idea used by the brain. Thinking is the medium used both negatively and positively, designed to create your experiences. You direct your thinking.

Therefore, it is important to become skilled at managing your thoughts. You direct your thoughts, words and beliefs by using the "Boss", your inner life. Do you want to change your thoughts, words and beliefs by using the "Boss", your inner life? Do you want to change your body? Do you want a new weigh? Be inner directed, change your body, transform your life! You will learn how to be inner directed by practicing these exercises:

*Centered Personality Exercise*

Become very quiet, close your eyes, sit in a comfortable position where you will not be distracted by noise or people. Begin by letting go of all tension and stress, be quiet enough to feel your own heart beat, sense your pulse.

In the following exercise, you will be in a reflective state of awareness, open your eyes gently to read the ideas, and close between each section to follow instructions. Take as much time as you need. Have a pencil and paper ready for your responses. This exercise takes about 30 minutes the first time, about 10 to 15 minutes on a regular basis.

### Identification Dies-Identification

"We are dominated by everything with which the self becomes identified. We can dominate, direct and use everything from which we dis-identify ourselves." Dr. Roberto Assagioli

We are aware of and identify with three key components of our total self: the body, the intellect and emotions. When we identify with and focus our attention on a particular life component, this becomes the dominant expression of our lives. Many times we become so identified with that part of us that we think that it is who we are. An example of this identification can be seen in the athlete whose focus is on the body and the achievement attained through the body expression, you might hear, "this is my life." In order to express in total, we must dies-identify from a single focus.

You will realize, through the following exercise, that you, the "centered" you, are the observer. Because you cannot be both the observer and the observed, you can dis-identify from any object or experience that you are observing. For example, I have emotions, such as fear, but I am not that fear. I identify the fear as my experience but when I observe the fear, I realize that it is not me, only what I am observing and therefore experiencing. So I dis-identify

22

from it.  I can dis-identify from it by using a statement such as, "there is within me a state of fear but it is not me."

The observer is the dominant I, the "centered" I.  As the observer, I dominate and manage all the parts of my life.  The "centered" I is the Boss in the experience of getting over weight.  A statement regarding weight might be:  there is within me a state of extra weight, but it is not me, not who I am.

Your life is like a kaleidoscope.  All of the beautiful parts are there but inactive without a dominant operator.  The system only works when the operator works it.  The operator is the observer.  Without direction and choice, the operator only makes scattered patterns or pictures.  So it is with you.  You are the dominant operator, the observer in your own life.  You choose the patterns and expressions of life that become your experience.  You, the centered you, are the operator of your life, you are the "Boss."

> Note:  This concept is a psychological (metaphysical) concept.
> You may need to read it several times for clarity.

Now do the following exercise:

### Identification / Dis-identification Exercise

### Body

I have a body.  I am aware of my body at many levels, sensations and feelings.  I am aware of my breath.  As I take it in, I can feel it coming into my body; as I exhale, I feel that warmth of air.  I sense my heartbeat, beating in rhythm, pulsating at my throat, temples, and wrists.  I can feel different sensations in my body, where it is comfortable and uncomfortable.  I inquire, who is aware, who is the observer of my body?  I have a body, but I am not my body.  My body serves as a place for me to live, a temple where life resides; a package, a gift, but it is not me.  I have a body but I am not my body.

### Intellect

I have an intellect.  I can hear, picture and dream in thoughts, words and ideas.  Sometimes when the thoughts seem to overpower me, I want to slow down my thoughts.  Sometimes I feel confused, at times it appears that I cannot stop thinking about a situation, idea, challenge, song or person.  Ordinarily we identify ourselves with our thoughts.  When we observe ourselves while we think we notice that the intellect works like an instrument. When I replace the thoughts with another thought, I do it on purpose or consciously. Therefore, I have a thinking brain, but I am not that brain. I can observe, direct, and change it when I choose. I have use of it but it is not who I am. I am not my intellect. I have a brain but I am not my intellect.

## Emotions

I have emotions, but I am not my emotions. My emotions are like waves, sometimes high, joyous, excited, and expectant; other times low, fearful, anxious and worried. I am sometimes jealous and competitive. My emotions are cooperating, comparing and living, but when I choose to change them I can. I have emotions, but I am not my emotions. Yes, I can use emotions to measure my feelings and indicate what responses to give, but they are not me, myself. I am not my emotions, I observe them and choose the appropriate responses, but they are not me.

What then is left of my personal components if I am not body, mind or emotions? It is the essence of who I am, the life within, called my "centered" self. I can feel this life within me as an observer. When I am in tune with this life within, I gain control and management of my life. It is my presence, my essence-my own uniqueness.

The inner image exercise, that you have completed, allows you to communicate with your higher self and make decisions based on that communication. It allows you to build an image for your own body; your own unique image of what your body can be, not the world's, but your own.

The physical condition and shape of your body is your choice. Our bodies demonstrate choices through our thoughts, our beliefs. Your present body is a direct reflection of the beliefs you hold about it. It is our mind that creates the physical reality that we experience, especially evident in the form of our body. If you do not have a constructive, clear image of how you want your body to feel and look, it will and must "embody" your unconscious beliefs.

It is important that you communicate with your body every day during this 21 day experience. Sit in a quiet, comfortable place and commune with your body. Ask it questions and as it responds to you, listen and follow to the letter what you hear. How will you know it is your own higher self speaking and not just random thoughts? The higher thoughts are always positive, never critical or judgmental. The ideas feel "right."

Ask your body these and/or your own questions.  Respond from your inner self.

1.  What are the things that make life satisfying?

2.  Am I satisfied with my body now?

3.  What do I want to achieve with reference to body, health and weight?

4.  What have I already achieved that makes me proud with reference to body, health and weight?

5.  What makes me a beautiful person?  Make a list.

6.  What have I done to make my body healthy?  How do I feel about this?

7.  What is my physical condition?  Am I in good condition?  In what ways?

8.  In what ways am I not in good health?

9.  Are my circulatory, respiratory, neurological, cardiovascular and digestive systems in order?  Where do I need help?

10. How supple and flexible is my body?  How do I feel about this and what can be done to help?

11. Do you like the foods I put into you?  What are the foods you like, that are good for you, and what foods don't you like?

12. What are the foods you are allergic or sensitive to?

13. Do you enjoy my eating schedule?  Be specific?  What should my eating schedule be?

14. Do you get enough exercise?  What kind of exercise will be best for you?  How often?

15. Are you getting an appropriate amount of sleep or rest?  How many hours rest do you need to function at a high level?

16. What vitamins, minerals or supplements do you need to complete your nutritional program? Be specific.

17. Do you have any fears related to your body or health?

18. Do you feel loved? How do you feel about this?

19. In what ways can this love be expressed?

20. Do you have anything else you would like to tell me?

21. Describe your ideal body in detail; picture it every day.

# Day 2
## Part II:  Get Into The Rhythm Of Life

All of life works in rhythm. It happens in order. If You are eating out of order, your body and weight will reflect it. The body grows, maintains and balances itself in three life rhythm cycles: intake (take in food), assimilate (use food), and eliminate (release waste). When you move and act in rhythm with these cycles you will be healthy and enjoy a perfect body image.

When you learn to eat on schedule, your body will respond. Your body works by pattern and reacts to what your mind directs it to do. If you eat out of time, the body goes into protection of itself. If you do not eat for one or two meals, the body, because of its intelligence, feels that it is going into starvation, into ketosis, and therefore holds the next meal in storage. People who eat out of rhythm in this pattern don't coordinate the metabolic system as the body does not know what to expect or how to protect itself. This cycle is the one sure way of giving and holding fat in storage.

When you eat regular small meals in body rhythm, your body will use the calories as energy, burn them, eliminate them and you will lose or maintain *your own* healthy weight. In other words, this is the weight that is best for you.

# Day 2
## Part III:          Transform Your Spirit

### Be Conscious of Who You Are, Experience the "Ah Ha."

Component number two of the transformation model is to become conscious, awake to your beliefs, your words and actions. Being alert and present to what you are doing and being will allow you to choose, direct and create the life styles and experiences that contribute to your success in releasing weight. Do you look at yourself and say, "I'm fat, I don't look my best, I'm ugly, my health is bad," and so forth? These are thoughts that you have made logical because of what you are focusing your attention on, practicing, what you believe is true.

Your inner "I" dictates who you are. Be conscious of the patterns of your life. You have set up habits, feelings and an environment that support your body as it is today. What you experience as real in your body, your life is what you are conscious of as your truth. You say, "but if you could see me you would agree, I'm fat... This may be real, but it is not your truth. —If we were looking at a rainbow we would both agree that it is real, right? The rainbow is a reflection of a physical reality, like the mirage of wet pavement on the road on a hot day. These physical forms are real but they are not truth. They are reality created and/or affected by the environment, a physical coincidence. So you too are changed by your mental environment, which causes the physical coincidences or patterns that appear real to you. Can you transform your body? You bet you can.

Yes, change your thoughts, attitudes and actions about it. Remember, your body is in your mind, not as we have formerly been taught to believe, that your mind is somehow housed in your body. What is housed in your body is a brain. A brain is an organ used by the nervous system and the intellect. Make this theory logical by remembering the multiple personality psychology. Where the mind goes, the body follows.

You can help make your new goals logical by looking at pictures, visions and symbols of your ideal self. Keep your vision clear, see your image as true for you See yourself as this new image every day. Observe others who have transformed their bodies. If anyone can do it, you can. Keep believing in the answers; do not put your attention on the problem. Your problems are not you; you have created them out of your beliefs. You can un-create them out of your beliefs. Be conscious of who you are, wake up, feel the success.

**Exercise** (Indoors for 30 Minutes)
Jog for fun: Jog in place while watching your favorite show.

Insight

Action

**Affirmation**

*My attention to anything is practicing it, whatever I practice I become good at.*
*My full attention is on transforming my life in a new weigh, I.* love myself.

# Menu Options
## "Fuel For the Day" - "Hectic Day"

---

**BREAKFAST**

Creamy P.B. & J.:

1 tablespoon Laura Scudder's Natural peanut butter

1 tablespoon ricotta cheese made with skim milk

2 teaspoons Smucker's Simply Fruit jam (100% fruit, no sugar)

1 slice of whole wheat bread

---

*Spread peanut butter, cheese and jam on whole wheat bread. Enjoy one cup cubed cantaloupe on the side.*

**Snack Boost**

2 dried apricots

3 unsalted almonds

*(in a Zip-loc snack bag)*

---

**LUNCH**

Turkey Sandwich:

2 slices of fresh unsalted turkey

½ teaspoon of mustard

Lettuce and tomato

Between 2 slices of whole wheat bread

Fruit

---

**Snack**

Fruit

---

**DINNER**

Bean and Cheese Burrito:

¼ cup Rosarita fat-free refried beans

½ cup chopped cooked chicken

1 tablespoon low-fat shredded cheese

1 whole wheat tortilla

---

*Spoon beans into tortilla. Sprinkle cheese on top of beans. Roll up tortilla. Heat in microwave for 2 minutes on high. Have a salad on the side with one tablespoon fat-free salad dressing.*

**Snack**

Cream Cheese Rice Cake and Jam:

1 plain unsalted rice cake topped with:

1 tablespoon Philadelphia Light cream cheese

1 teaspoon Smucker's Simply Fruit jam (100% fruit, no sugar)

***Your day was:*** Approximately 1,234 calories, 1,889 mg. sodium, 118 mg. cholesterol

24% protein          55% carbohydrates          21% fat

# Day 3

**Part I:**    **You Are What You Think**

**Part II:**    **Body By Design**

**Part III:**    **Image in Action – Spells Imagination**

**Just For You (Your Own Uniqueness)**

Create a new look for yourself, a hairstyle, a flair of color in your hair or a cut, wear something daring. If you've never worn shorts, try it. Get a new hairdo, give yourself a makeover--better yet, have one done.

# Day 3
## Part I:                       You Are What You Think

Yesterday you began an exciting journey in your life. Today the adventure continues. Looking into your inner attitudes was a turning point. Through self-awareness you have begun to create an entirely new dimension in your thinking and your life.

You are now, to some extent, aware that your thinking is your life. You are where you are now because of your thinking. For example, your thinking led you to this experience because you are thinking of change. Similarly, your thinking led you to your present life. Now thinking will move you to the richer, more rewarding life you desire, free from weighting.

You will get as much out of life as you think.

Life has an unlimited amount of success, happiness, joy and fulfillment waiting for you. All you have to do is think about these things, put them into action, and they will come to pass. You can experience abundance if you think of abundance. Of course, if you think of lack, that is what you experience. You experience abundance only to the degree that you recognize and accept it. Even if abundance is not real to you, think of it as real, and it will become real. You create what is real. You define reality. You weave it. Look at yourself and see that you are what you think. Thought is the tool that created your limitations, thought will create your life anew.


# Day 3
## Part II:                       Body By Design

The American standard for good looks calls for a supple, proportioned, slender, but properly rounded, body. How do you fit this image? How do you know if you are slender enough, or round enough? Who determines the standard?

Sixty-one percent of the population in the United States claim to be overweight. What is your I.Q? In other words, what is your image quotient? How does your image measure up? Experts in recent studies have found that Americans have an "ideal" image of the perfect man or woman. However, the perfect person has not been defined necessarily by any one entity, one group or person, but is marketed across the screens of T.V. and movies, pictured in magazine ads and displayed on billboards. Americans are obsessed with the "Image Myths." You are required to have this mythical image to get a job, to have friends, to get married or climb the career "ladder of success."

Inappropriate concern about weight and personal approval has caused people to go to such extremes as anorexia nervosa, bulimia and other eating disorders in order to fit the commercial image quotient or I.Q. You need not measure up to the Madison Avenue Myth. It is time you explore who you are. It is time to discover your unique body design.

### Body Design Exercise

Each of us is born with a body design. This design is sometimes related to genetics, as are your inherited features, such as general looks, height, or color. Throughout history, health authorities have identified bodies as types. In America these types are known as:

1. Endomorph-a body type that is slender, having fast-acting thyroid and metabolism
2. mesomorph-medium build, average stamina
3. obese-heavy, slow digestion, deliberate, slow metabolism

These body types dictate the amount of food you can eat, how you assimilate the food you eat, your health and temperament.

There is an ancient Indian medical science dating back more than 6,000 years, called Ayurveda. Ayurveda comes from the Sanskrit root words, Ayur or life, and Veda, meaning knowledge or science. Ayurveda is a proven life science. This science states that our body types or designs are like blue prints, outlining our innate tendencies. They indicate the basic components of our system. Knowing your body design is essential to understanding yourself and managing your weight and health. Every time an event happens in the mind there is a corresponding event that happens in the body. Mind and body correlate in every way. Therefore, it is imperative that we know our body design. Example, fear can make you sweat, have diarrhea, or lose sleep, all affecting the body, appetite and digestion. Where is the fear? It's in your mind; of course.

What if you could have the body you have always dreamed of, not society's version, but your version? What would it look like? Have you ever really thought about that? Your thoughts create your body. There is nowhere that the concept of mind and body is more visible than with our bodies.

Everyone has the same kind of cells, organs and systems. Despite the variations from one personality to the next, we also share the same range of emotions. What makes each of us express a different blueprint or body design? Ayurveda says the answer lies in the meeting point between mind and body. How we think and what we think determines our body. Clearly the two do meet and where they do thoughts turn into matter. This principle operates through these body designs.

These are metabolic principles connecting the mind and body. They allow the mind to dialog and talk to the body. Every thought, emotion, hope, or fear leaves its mark on the body. These mental events constantly shape the body as they "talk" to it. The body designs need to be recognized and trained so that you can benefit physically by the mind - body connection. The three body designs are called vata, pitta, and kapha. Get an idea of your body design by completing the body design form. Remember, you are a combination of all of these, but one is dominant.

Vata - controls movement
Pitta - controls metabolism
Kapha - controls structure

## Body Design Quiz

|  | Vata | Pitta | Kapha |
|---|---|---|---|
| Type of hair | ☐ Dry | ☐ Fine, thinning, reddish, prematurely gray | ☐ Thick, oil |
| Skin | ☐ Dry, rough | ☐ Soft, ruddy | ☐ Oily, moist |
| Mental activity | ☐ Quick mind, restless, imaginative | ☐ Sharp intellect, efficient, perfectionist | ☐ Calm, steady, stable |
| Memory | ☐ Quick to learn, quick to forget | ☐ Good general memory | ☐ Good long-term memory |
| Weather | ☐ Aversion to cold weather | ☐ Aversion to hot weather | ☐ Aversion to damp, cool weather |
| Sleep | ☐ Interrupted, light sleep | ☐ Sound, medium sleep time | ☐ Heavy sleeper |

| | Vata | Pitta | Kapha |
|---|---|---|---|
| Reaction to stress | ☐ Excites easily, anxious, worried | ☐ Angers easily, irritated, critical | ☐ Not easily ruffled, stubborn |
| Friendship | ☐ Make friends easily | ☐ Occupation-related, slow to make friends | ☐ Long-lasting friendships |
| Weight | ☐ Hard to gain | ☐ Average weight | ☐ Gain easily |
| Hunger | ☐ Irregular | ☐ Regular meals | ☐ Can skip meals |
| Walk | ☐ Quick | ☐ Determined | ☐ Slow, steady |
| Would like to change | ☐ Worry | ☐ Intensity | ☐ Depression |
| Moods | ☐ Changeable | ☐ Slow to modify | ☐ No change |
| Totals | | | |

*The following activities can help you to stay in charge:*

Vata (out of balance):

Worry
Fasting (eating)
Do not get enough sleep
Eat on the run
Keep no routine whatsoever
Eat dry, frozen or leftover foods
Run around a lot
Never lubricate your skin
Work the graveyard shift
Avoid tranquil, warm, moist places
Uses drugs, especially cocaine and speed
Have major abdominal surgery
Repress your feelings

Vata (in balance):

Keep warm
Choose home-cooked food
Avoid cold foods/drinks
Minimize eating raw foods
take it easy on the beans
Drink lots of water
Emphasize sweet, sour, salty
Keep routine
Live in secure environment

Pitta (out of balance):

Drink plenty of alcohol
Eat spicy foods
Engage in frustrating activities
Emphasize tomatoes, chilies, raw onions; sour foods

Pitta (in balance):

keep cool
Avoid excess heat, humidity
Avoid excess oil, fried foods
avoid salt, red meat, spices

Exercise at the hottest time of the day
Wear tight, hot clothes
Use drugs, especially cocaine, speed or marijuana
Avoid cool, fresh, peaceful places
Snack on highly salted foods
Repress your feelings
Eat as much red meat and salted fish as possible

Avoid alcohol, drugs
Eat fresh fruits, vegetables
Drink milk, cheese, grains
Get fresh air
Trust your feelings

Kapha (out of balance):

Take nice long naps after meals
Eat lots of fatty foods and oils
minimum
Overeat as often and as much as possible
Deny your creative self
Luxuriate in inertia
Become a couch potato
Assume someone else will do it
Avoid invigorating; warm, dry areas
Do not exercise
Live on potato chips and beer
Use drugs, especially sedatives and tranquilizers
Repress your feelings
Make sure you get at least one dessert every day

Kapha (in balance):

get plenty of physical activity
Keep consumption of fat to

Avoid cold foods, sweets, breads
Choose warm, light, dry foods
Minimize liquids (except water)
Emphasize pungent, bitter and
    astringent tastes
luxuriate in fresh vegetables, herbs
    and spices
Get enough complex carbohydrates
Allow excitement, challenge and
    change in your life

# Day 3
# Part III:      Image in Action - Spells Imagination

Step three of the transformation model is taking action. You know what you want. You must create the plan of action, set goals. Look at ways you can change the old behavior. You already know that what you put your attention on becomes your experience. You cannot think of peaches and lemons at the same time. When you look at your body it demonstrates to you that you have moved it out of balance and many times out of line with reference to discipline. This is because you are letting the body control you instead of it being managed by the centered self, the "I," the "Boss." You must take action to discipline your affairs and your behavior not out of judgment but love.

Image thinking is thinking beyond the appearance of self created boundaries. Do you know any image thinkers? Columbus was one, turns out the world is round. Einstien's relativity, Col. Sander's fried chicken. Who do you know, personally who has stepped beyond the impossible? You are probably one of them.. Ever remember someone telling you what you couldn't do? Yeah!

This is the most challenging component in the transformation model. Keep believing in the answers; do not put your attention on the problems. You have done it that way and it hasn't worked. You must unlock the door of your mind, image plus action does it.

*Exercise:* (indoors 30 minutes)

*Run for fun*: Jog in place while watching a TV show (commercials, too)

*Insight:*

*Action:*

*Affirmation:*
Gratitude is my practice, not my motto.

# Menu Options
## "Fuel For the Day" - "Good for Craving-Salt Day"

---
**BREAKFAST**

Hot Apple Oatmeal:

| | |
|---|---|
| 1 cup cooked plain oatmeal | 2 teaspoons 100% all fruit jam |
| ½ cup skim or low-fat milk | ½ cup diced apple |
| ½ teaspoon cinnamon | |

---

*Cut up apple and cook in microwave until soft and warm.  Heat up oatmeal and put in jam to sweeten.  Top oatmeal with cooked apples, cinnamon and milk.*

**Snack**

Celery with Peanut Butter:

2 stalks of celery, each stalk filled with 2 teaspoons Laura Scudder's unsalted natural peanut butter

---
**LUNCH**

Healthy Guacamole:

| | |
|---|---|
| 2-ounce slice of avocado | 1/8 cup diced tomatoes |
| ½ cup non-fat cottage cheese | Salsa to taste |
| 1 slice whole wheat tortilla | |

*Mash the avocado with the cottage cheese and stir in diced tomatoes and salsa.  Place on top of warmed whole wheat tortilla.  Eat with a vegetable or fruit.*

---

**Snack**

Cheesy Corn Puffs:

1 cup puffed corn (in bag in market, cereal section, brand name "Pure & Simple" or "El Molino"--ingredients should say only "whole corn")

1 tablespoon fat-free grated Parmesan cheese

*Put puffed corn and Parmesan cheese in a paper bag and shake.*

---
**DINNER**

Sloppy Susan:

¼ cup ground turkey

¼ cup tomato sauce

1 teaspoon chili powder

1/8 cup diced onions

1 whole wheat hamburger bun

---

*Brown onions and ground turkey in non-stick pan.  Add tomato sauce and simmer for 5 minutes.  Serve over open-faced hamburger bun with a salad.*

**Snack**

Veggies & Dip:

Cut up raw mushrooms, broccoli, carrots, etc.  Heat up Rosarita refried beans.  Dip vegetables in dip.

***Your day was:***    Approx. 1,268 calories, 2,111 mg. sodium, and 79 mg. cholesterol

| | | |
|---|---|---|
| 23% protein | 51% carbohydrates | 26% fat |

# Day 4

**Part I:**       **Image Myths**

**Part II:**     **Image In Yourself**

**Part III:**    **You Are The Example of Your Action**

**Just For You (<u>Y</u>our <u>O</u>wn <u>U</u>niqueness)**

Get out the family album, look at the pictures and feel the pride your family memories bring.  It is fun to reminisce.

# Day 4
## Part I:                                   Image Myths

Heredity has dealt all of us certain body structures and features which differ from body design and over which we have no control. We come in various packages--tall, short, large or small boned, wide or narrow hipped. No one is surprised when tall people have tall children. However, if you are large, the assumption is that you got that way solely because you fell into one of many "fat people" stereotypes. These stereotypes are image myths. Some of these myths are lack of will, laziness, low self-esteem and many more. Make no mistake; your genes are not necessarily responsible for the fat on your body. Environment, behavior and modeling are some contributors. Your bone structure and body design are heredity factors. So, if you are a member of a family of large-proportioned people take note and work with those features to look your very best. Take a look at your family tree and do not try to make an apple tree from an orange seed.

Although your basic framework cannot be changed, you can change the padding around your bones to produce your best look. Anyone, whether ideally proportioned or not, looks best when the body is smooth and firm.

Personal transformation comes from positive affirmation. You must dispel the negative image myths, change them to positive affirmations. Eat healthy, breathe deeply, exercise and express rhythm with life, listen to your centered self, follow its direction and create your own perfect body proportions. You can choose the body proportions that you feel happy with, rather than leaving the choice to the myths and standards set by TV commercials, magazines, family and friends. A healthy body is the foundation of your personal success. If you are going along with negative myths, it affects your work, your dependability, your attitude and your overall energy. Your total image depends largely on the way you feel about your body. Do not complain about being overweight; give yourself permission to get over it once and for all. No one wants to hear the old myths; no one wants to come to your pity party, with the repetition of all the same old affirmations served. If you shouldn't eat this or that and you are going to eat it anyway, do not announce to the world that you are not going to choose, that you are a victim. Be mature enough to manage your life. You may enjoy being the victim. Listen to the "Boss"; you will tell yourself what is best for you. Listen, listen, and listen.

# Image Myths and Negative Programming

Your behavior is largely determined by what you see or imagine as truth. These images are created from the words you use. You think in words; you lay out your life by words; you tend to be governed by the words with which you talk to yourself. A hypnotist can control a subject's physical reactions merely by words. You are really doing the same to yourself. You have spent all of your life hypnotizing yourself. Every word you repeat and believe tends to shape what you become.

Let's look at some words you use that might be having a negative effect on your life. These are called image myths. They're really negative affirmations.

Image Myths are words you feed into your mind that shape your attitudes. Once you plant these myths into your mind, they become fact. The mind is like a garden. It will grow any kind of seeds you plant in it. The image myths are negative seeds that take root and grow. The image myths below are sentences written down by others who have participated in the "New Weigh" experience:

1. How many apply to you?

2. What Image Myths are you using that are not listed? How are they affecting your life? Your self-confidence? How can image myths affect your health? Your success? Your relationship with others? Your weight/image?

3. Image Myths are negative affirmations. What positive affirmations can you use to eliminate your Image Myths?
   "I'm so fat."
   "I'm too old to change."
   "I'm self-conscious."
   "I can't remember people's names."
   "I'll never be a rich person."
   "I can't lose weight."
   "I don't seem to have much patience."
   "I'm a procrastinator."
   "I never look good when I go out."
   "I worry a lot."
   "I can't get organized."
   "Cancer runs in my family."

## Changing Myths to Affirmations

On the space below, write the myths that you believe about yourself, your opportunities, and your limitations. On the other side, write an affirmation that counteracts the myth.

| Myth | Affirmation |
|------|-------------|
|      |             |

# Day 4
## Part II:  "Image-In" (Imagine) Yourself

Your appearance, how you package yourself, tells a story--make it tell the right story. You have an opportunity to present your other qualifications... later. It's the first four seconds of a personal encounter that create a first impression, so do not forget the adage that "You may not have a second chance to make the first impression." Health, vitality, grooming, carriage, makeup, body proportions, hair style and overall "good looks" make a statement about how you care for yourself in those first crucial moments.

Image is your inner face, but it is also what you see outside. It is your personal visualization in outer expression. You express what you conceive yourself to be. Your mind does not differentiate between a real image and an imagined one. This allows you to make your imagined image the real one. The secret of creating the image you have always wanted is to visualize it (see it, imagine it), think, feel, and act as if the image you want is the image you have. You must completely submerge yourself in this new image; you must live it out to the full. If you do this, you will resculpt that inner face created by your responses to past events. Your new inner face will actively produce your new outer image, step by step. Build a beautiful package, a powerful presence, through this 21-day experience. To build your presence is to practice bringing forth your own unique expression.

You are whatever you believe yourself to be right now. Do not harass your subconscious with negative opinions; nurture it with positive feelings and it will fortify your resolve and success in the world.

### Exercise:

You have probably discovered through your own experiences that your self-image has been rather haphazardly developed by the events in your past. Now consider your goals for your new package. On a sheet of paper list the qualities and characteristics of the ideal you.

Look at yourself.

Do you like what you see? Look at your inner self, your personality, the way you think. Look at your outer self, your body, your environment. Do you feel close to your ideal self? Is the total you all that you desire to be? If you feel you can be more, much more, then put pen to paper and draw two columns. In one column write out the real you. In the other, write out the ideal you. Before you have finished the experience, you will move toward making the ideal you, the real you. The image is in you already. Image-in (imagine) yourself!

# Day 4
# Part III:    You Are the Example of Your Action

The fourth component of the transformation model is to consciously act out  what you desire to transform  I consciously (on purpose) act like I am beautiful. I dress, walk, talk in my best form. I use my best manners. I respond to life with poise and grace in all situations and to all people. Wherever I go, I act as if it is the most important occasion of my life and I am going to meet the most important people. I act like the beautiful person that I am. I live, move and have my being in these new truths about me. I am the example of my actions. The fourth step of the transformation model is making your actions conscious ones. Be aware of your new behavior at all times. Be on purpose, it works!

### Exploring My Body Image

Developing a positive healthy body image is very important as we learn to make new lifestyle changes and bring our weight within an appropriate range.

1.    What words or phrases do I currently use to describe my body?

2.    How has my body image come to be this way?

3.   How do negative feelings and attitudes surrounding my body affect my life
     In general.

4.   What can I do to change this response?

Changing the negative body image requires an acceptance of who you are.  Learn
to respect yourself unconditionally.  Accept the fact that your body is yours and
you are working toward improvement.  It is not the same as resignation where
you give in and give up.  Acceptance will give you the potential to move beyond
where you are.

*We cannot change anything unless we accept it.  Condemnation does not
liberate, it oppresses. "*

                                        Carl Gustav Jung

*Exercise:* (indoors, 20 minutes)

*Stretch and flex.* Do floor exercises. Stretch, do leg lifts, extensions, arm reaches, bend, stoop.

**Insight/Action:**

<u>Insight</u>:

<u>Action</u>:

**Affirmation:**

Only those who will risk going too far... can possible find out how far one can go.

# Menu Options
## "Fuel For the Day"

---

**BREAKFAST**

Egg Burrito:

| | |
|---|---|
| ½ cup Eggbeaters | Diced tomatoes |
| 1 tablespoon cheese | Vegetable spray |
| Salsa to taste | Whole wheat tortilla |

---

*Scramble up Eggbeaters in non-stick pan sprayed with vegetable spray (e.g., Pam). Put in tortilla on top of Eggbeaters while cooking. Put top on fry pan for a few seconds ((to heat tortilla). Put tortilla on a plate filled with Eggbeaters, cheese and tomatoes. Add salsa to taste. Eat a fruit to balance this meal (grapefruit, orange, cantaloupe, etc.).*

**Snack Boost**

2 dried apricots
3 unsalted almonds
*(In a Zip-loc snack bag)*

---

**LUNCH**

Curried Chicken Stuffed Potato:

| | |
|---|---|
| ½ cup diced cooked chicken | ¼ cup cooked peas |
| 1 medium potato | ¼ cup yogurt |
| 1 tsp. tumeric | 1 tsp. curry |

*Cook potato in microwave until soft. Fill with chicken and peas and heat again. Cover with yogurt and seasonings and heat for a few more seconds. Have a salad on the side.*

---

**Snack**

Cottage Cheese and Fruit
½ cup non-fat cottage cheese
1 cup grapes

---

**DINNER**

Spaghetti with Meat Sauce:
¾ cup whole wheat pasta
¼ cup cooked ground turkey
¼ cup spaghetti sauce (Classico or Bertolli), all vegetable, and no meat

---

*Cook pasta in a sauce pan. Drain and top with heated spaghetti sauce and cooked ground turkey. Eat 1 cup vegetables on the side.*

**Snack**

Chocolate Soy Shake:
½ cup Westsoy Lite chocolate soy milk mixed in blender with ½ banana, until bubbly.

***Your day was:*** Approximately 1,268 calories, 2,111 mg. sodium, and 79 mg. cholesterol

| | | |
|---|---|---|
| 23% protein | 51% carbohydrates | 26% fat |

# Day 5

**Part I:**       **One Day At A Time**

**Part II:**     **Take A Breath**

**Part III:**    **Practice, Practice, Practice**

## Just For You (<u>Y</u>our <u>O</u>wn <u>U</u>niqueness)

Write a positive affirmation (statement with which you agree). Write it on a card; put it on your refrigerator, or wherever you can see it, to remind yourself that you are the best friend you can have. Example: <u>I am my own best friend.</u>

# Day 5:
## Part I:                    One Day At A Time

Information is power.  Power is the ability to affect change.  You have a right to expect success.  Give yourself the right to process this information day by day, one day at a time.  Give yourself the right to set up your new schedule.  Give yourself the gift of setting up your new plan.  Do it one day at a time and it becomes simple.  Remember the old adage, "By the yard it's hard, by the inch it's a cinch."  When you direct your life today, that's all you need.  After all, you only have the present moment, today.  It is written that yesterday is a dream, tomorrow a vision.  Today, well lived, makes every day a vision of hope.  Plan, set up the food schedules you need.  Inventory and shop for the food you need, and then you will not be left unprepared.  There are no fake foods or crazy ingredients to find.  You have no gimmicks to learn, only sensible, enjoyable living.  Be aware of how good you feel, how your image changes and what made that happen.  The actions and behavior that you have chosen help you and are easy to do.  You've made it happen.  Enjoy today and tomorrow will take care of itself.

# Day 5
## Part II:                    Take A Breath

1.    Breath is life.  From the first faint breath of the newborn infant, to the last gasp of the dying, life is a series of breaths.

2.    Breathing is life's most important function and when we stop to think of it-- few of us give any thought to the breath, however--we find that all of our bodily functions are dependent upon our breath.

3.    It certainly is not necessary to explore why we need to breathe.  This is self-evident, but how we breathe is not.  We usually take very shallow, short breaths, as though there is a limited amount for each of us.  It is vital that we get enough breath; it is the food of life.  Correct breathing is so important.  It is the channel through which physical perfection comes to us.

4.	Breath is power. Everything is in the air. Radio, today, can project sound seven and a half times around the earth in a second, carrying sound at the inconceivable speed of light. What transports this power? It is called ether and it is everywhere in the atmosphere. The same powerful ether is the air that we breathe.

5.	With proper breathing your physical appearance changes. Your mental capacities sharpen. It is food for your mind and body.

***Breathing Exercise Upon Rising (do not strain)***

- Sit or stand erect; see the spine as straight, posture erect
- Breathe deeply, inhaling for sixteen counts, one nostril at a time
- Exhale for sixteen counts -- do this inhale/exhale exercise four times in the morning, at noon and at night. Inhale life energy, exhale toxins and anxiety. Release all stress and receive the life-giving substance of air. It activates your metabolism to assist you in burning fat.

# Day 5
# Part III:	Practice, Practice, Practice

Become conscious that you are acting beautifully. The fifth process of transformation takes practice, practice, practice. When I think I look fat, I must see myself as toned and healthy instead. Run your hands down your body and say, "Thank you for housing me and being your best self at all times" (it is true that the body is doing its best now). Say to your body, "I love you just the way you are."

You will practice consciously by listening to your centered "I, the Boss," and following its directions when it comes to food intake, drink, exercise, attitude, and action. Let go of the phrases "my body," "my fat," "my size," "my looks," as if they are a possession that you own. If we do not want to own the old self, let go of it lovingly, with no condemnation or judgment, by accepting the new loved one. I love myself right now. I am a beautiful, radiant expression of life. I know that to succeed I must practice, practice, practice. The more you practice, the more your new behavior will become routine, a habit. You will begin to act this way unconsciously. Your new image is synthesized (integrated) into your whole being. The fourth step is accomplished. You move from conscious practice to new unconscious behavior and you won't know when it happened, it just did.

.

*Exercise:* (indoors, 20 minutes)

   *Do salsa dancing, olé!* Put on the Latin sounds and move. Feel the drums, the intense passion in the music, express it!

*Insight/Action:*

Insight:

Action:

*Affirmation:*

   Enjoy your achievements as well as your dreams.

# Menu Options
## "Fuel For the Day"

---

**BREAKFAST**

Cheesy Fruity Danish:

1 tablespoon Knudsen's non-fat cottage cheese
1 tablespoon non-fat mozzarella cheese, shredded
1 tablespoon ricotta cheese made from skim milk
2 teaspoons 100% fruit jam (no sugar added)
¼ cup sliced apples, grapes, blueberries or strawberries
1 whole wheat English muffin

---

*Top split English muffin with cottage cheese and fruit and top with shredded mozzarella cheese. Place in the broiler oven until brown and bubbly.*

**Snack**

Fruit

---

**LUNCH**

Bean and Cheese Burrito:

½ cup Rosarita fat-free refried beans
1 tablespoon low-fat shredded cheddar cheese
1 whole wheat tortilla

---

*Spoon beans into tortilla. Sprinkle cheese on top of beans. Roll up tortilla. Heat in microwave for 2 minutes on high. Have a fruit or vegetable with this meal.*

**Snack**

2 dried apricots
3 unsalted almonds
*(in a Zip-loc snack bag)*

---

**DINNER**

Halibut and Rice:

4 ounces halibut (baked with lemon and Mrs. Dash)
½ cup cooked brown rice
Piquant Sauce to go over Halibut and Rice:
2 tablespoons catsup, low sodium
1 teaspoon mustard
2 tablespoons celery, diced
*Mix piquant ingredients in a bowl. Heat in microwave. Pour over Halibut and Rice.*
1 cup vegetables as a side dish.

---

**Snack**

Blueberry Cream Cheese Parfait:

1 cup blueberries (fresh or frozen)          2 tablespoons Cool Whip Lite
1 tablespoon Philadelphia Light cream cheese  1 teaspoon vanilla
*Fold together all ingredients and serve in a bowl. Makes 1 serving.*

---

***Your day was:***      Approximately 1,065 calories, 1,807 mg. sodium, 63 mg. cholesterol
                        22% protein          61% carbohydrates          17% fat

51

# Day 6

## Just For You (Your Own Uniqueness)

Have or give yourself a pedicure. Better yet, have a pedi-party with a friend or a special person. Soak your feet together in a tub and then give each other a pedicure. What a great sharing time.

# Day 6
## Part I:        Get In Touch With Yourself

To really get in touch with other people, you must first get in touch with yourself. This means that you must understand how you react to situations. You must, in other words, know the basis for your own emotional reactions. We sometimes behave in regrettable ways when our emotions are in control. Resentment, for example, is an emotion that is in control when we allow holding on to hurt feelings to persist, when we are not willing to take responsibility.

You first learned "what" to feel when you were a child. As many as 15,000 "No's" and "Can'ts" were impressed upon you when you were a child. You were punished, restricted and restrained. It is no wonder that you have some feelings of negative images and immaturity. You were dominated by adults who were twice as big. In relations with others, you could have felt frustrated, inferior, shy, and often, fearful. You faced many challenges as a child by crying, running or displaying tantrums and sulking. Another side of you learned "how" to feel. Your curiosity, laughter, enjoyment, creativity, imagination, and daring arose from your unrestricted child ego state. So, now, as a grown up, you have developed both positive, healthy, natural emotions that are free and child-like and negative, unhealthy and "educated" emotions that are restrictive. We sometimes give power to these negative emotions, which elicit childish responses and manipulative actions. "I want it.right now, I deserve it and I am going to have it." Sound familiar?

By becoming aware of your early programming, you realize that there is little that is productive about inappropriate emotions. Fear, impatience, frustration, jealousy, selfishness, anxiety and tension can be expressed inappropriately. Think about an experience of fear, take a moment to sort out the emotion, take a deep breath. You cannot help it if inappropriate emotions crop up, as they will from time to time, but tell yourself that they will not manipulate or control you, your thoughts, or your actions. Say to yourself, "I cannot help the way I feel right now, but I can help the way I think and act." Get in touch with your feelings. Take responsibility for your actions; go to your centered self, "the Boss," for support in making decisions that are best for you.

**Day 6**
**Part II:** **Exercise is a Must:**
**Benefits of Aerobic/Cardio Exercise**

We know that aerobic/cardio exercise is essential to permanent weight management. It burns extra calories, builds muscle, reduces stored fat, decreases appetite, is a natural stimulant and cuts down on stress plus stress-related eating. These facts may be reason enough to convince you to create and maintain an exercise routine. But there are so many more physical and mental health benefits that result from aerobic/cardio exercise.

Probably the most important health benefit of exercise is a better cardiovascular system and the reduced risk of suffering a heart attack or stroke. Exercise can prevent or decrease high blood pressure concerns. Exercise raises high-density lipoproteins, the good blood fats, and lowers low-density lipoproteins, the bad blood fats.

Exercise often reduces low-back pain. It helps to manage the negative effects of osteoporosis or brittle-bone disease. Regular exercise can help regulate blood sugar and will prevent or improve some blood sugar problems like diabetes (high blood sugar) and hypoglycemia (low blood sugar). Exercise done in a safe manner will improve many joint problems. Cardio exercise can improve your strength and endurance, making your life fuller and enjoyable because you will be able to do more activities with ease. Youthful vigor is a bi-product of regular exercise. That got my attention.

The mental health benefits of exercise are substantial. Exercise calms the intensity of feelings of anxiety and stress. It also lifts the spirits from feelings of depression and boredom. These mental health benefits are to some extent the result of physiological changes in the body that begin to happen after you've been exercising for about 20 minutes. Neurotransmitters called endorphins are released, giving you pleasant, happy, energetic high feelings. But the lifts in your spirits when you're exercising regularly come from more than the endorphins. Following a regular exercise routine enhances the feelings of self-esteem and personal management of your life. You're on track, a little helps a lot.

# Day 6
## Part III:            Let Go, Just Be

If you practice an activity long enough, it becomes natural and you no longer need to do, or think about it purposely, you can just be. You find yourself listening to the "Boss," and eating healthy, enjoyable foods without feeling deprived. You begin to dress your best all the time. Casual or formal, you look your very best self. You begin to be your best self, emotionally, and gracefully accept others and see in them their best. You truly are transformed when you do not know you are being your new self. You have let go of fear, anxiety, competition, comparison and pain. You are just being you (Your Own Uniqueness). And so the sixth step is to release the idea of working on the new you. Accept it as yours. Let go…just be you.

*Exercise:* (indoors 20 minutes)
Have a stretch--do cat movements, progress to lion, then big dinosaur.

*Insight/Action:*

Insight:

Action:

*Affirmation: No one can make me feel inferior without my consent.*

I

# Menu Options
### "Fuel For the Day"

---

**BREAKFAST**
Healthy Egg Muffin:
½ cup Eggbeaters
1 tablespoon shredded cheddar cheese
1 sliced beefsteak tomato
1 whole wheat English muffin (split)
Pepper to taste

---

*Cook up Eggbeaters in nonstick pan (sprayed with vegetable spray). Sprinkle cheddar cheese on top of Eggbeaters. Toast English muffin. Top muffin with tomato, Eggbeaters and cheese, and enjoy. Have a fruit on the side.*

**Snack**
2 dried apricots
3 unsalted almonds
*(in a Zip-loc snack bag)*

---

**LUNCH**
Tuna Pita:
1 whole wheat pita bread
3 oz. tuna packed in water (drained)
1 tablespoon fat-free mayonnaise
Lettuce and tomato

---

*Mix tuna with mayonnaise. Fill pita with tuna mixture and lettuce and tomato.*

**Snack**
Celery with Peanut Butter:
2 stalks of celery, each stalk filled with 2 teaspoons Laura Scudder's unsalted natural peanut butter

---

**DINNER**
Chicken Cacciatore:
1 baked skinless chicken breast
½ cup cooked linguine
¼ cup meatless spaghetti sauce
*Pour spaghetti sauce over chicken and linguine. Enjoy a green salad on the side with 1 tablespoon low-fat salad dressing.*

---

**Snack**
Baked Apple:
1 apple with 2 teaspoons 100% fruit jam (no sugar) on top
*Cook in microwave until soft*

**Your day was:** Approximately 1,266 calories, 2,315 mg. sodium, and 138 mg. cholesterol

| 31% protein | 51% carbohydrates | 18% fat |
|---|---|---|

# Day 7

**Part I:**        **Action Does It**

**Part II:**      **Your Inner
Communication**

**Part III:**     **Accept Your Ideal Image**

## Just For You (Your Own Uniqueness)

Take a leisurely walk to a quiet, special place.  Pause to appreciate
the surroundings.  Listen to your thoughts.

# Day 7
## Part I:              Action Does It

Noble action comes from dreams.  When you want something that inflames your imagination, then you are moved to act.  Once desires have been kindled, they make you restless and you are moved to make the images in your mind manifest in the real world.

The ancient Greeks proclaimed that one of the great virtues was "action."

There is nothing as inspiring and motivating as a person of action.  On the other hand, a person of indecision and inertia fails to gain respect.

Down through the ages, famous philosophers have agreed that action, to make things happen, is what living is all about.  Sir William Asler said, "To know just what has to be done, and then do it, comprises the whole philosophy of practical life."

Only by taking action do you learn how to do things and only through action do you learn to live.  When action is stifled, people become frustrated and bitter.  They lose hope and power.  Action uplifts the spirit, for it is the means to bring our ideas into the world of expression.

Longfellow said, "Each morning see some task begun, each evening see it close, something attempted, something done has earned a night's repose."

# Day 7:
## Part II:     Your Inner Communion (meditation)

There are different concepts that are associated with the word meditation.  In a more restricted sense, it can be regarded as synonymous with disciplined thoughts or reflection on an idea.  On a broader, spiritual basis, it is simply the activity of silently listening to the spirit or higher self within.  Many people feel that meditation is only directed thought, or guided participation.  Actually there are three principle types of meditation:  reflective, receptive and creative.  All meditation is the activity of going beyond the noise in your head, beyond the thoughts to a place that is silent, peaceful and quiet. In this place you transcend sickness, fear, anxiety and other negative energies. The following is a brief overview of three types of meditation:

I. Reflective Meditation:

One simple definition is to think, an accurate but limited definition, since clear ideas or the function of thinking are not common property. The working of our mind normally proceeds spontaneously under the action of stimuli and interests of various kinds in a disorganized way. The mind operates independently of personal will and often is opposed to it. The lesson or focus of reflective meditation is to allow the thought to move in its own direction and observe and reflect on the messages.

II. Receptive Meditation:

Regard the mind as an inner friend and be ready to receive answers, ideas and revelations. How and in what form do the messages come? What material do we receive? The most common way is by vision or illumination. As has been said, the mind is symbolically an "inner eye" and therefore, it can become aware of the meaning of facts, events, decisions and solutions of problems. When we have an idea or a hunch, we are experiencing an intuition. We all can experience intuition. It is simply your intuition (in=inner; tuition=tutor), your inner teacher; listen to it.

III. Creative Meditation:

Meditation can be created because it is "inner action." There are various purposes for creative meditation. The first, and most important, is finding solutions, new paths. By means of meditation you can modify, transform and regenerate your personality. One effective way of doing this is by visualizing your ideal self, seeing this in quiet contemplative thought and developing a belief about it. Remember the ideal self includes physical, mental and emotional health based on spiritual unity and recognition of your identity.

What are the benefits of meditation?

☐ improves health and well being
☐ reduces high blood pressure
☐ stimulates intelligent thinking

□ reduces stress
□ assists in mental clarity
□ helps with sleep disorders
□ encourages creativity
□ increases the stability of the nervous system
□ improves resistance to disease
□ stabilizes emotions

As meditation deepens, compulsions, cravings and fits of emotion begin to lose their power to dictate your behavior. You see clearly that choices are possible. You will discover that the body is merely a garment you wear. You will know that you can manage your mind.

# Day 7
# Part III:        Accept Your Ideal Image

Act like the example of your new image. Help others by being well organized and happy. Display confidence without arrogance or inappropriate expanse of your ego. Express that this process works, that it is possible for anyone. Do not offer suggestions or guidance unless it is requested. Keep criticism, judgement, and comparison out of your life. If you judge or compare yourself with others, you will begin to transform the model again back to where you were because your attention and belief are on the negative.

You have learned to be free to choose, to release your own beautiful image, now you must accept this as so. See it in others too. Say to yourself, "I accept my freedom and the freedom of all others. I accept my ideal image. It is who I am."

*Exercise:*  (indoors 20 minutes)

Have a ball--use 6" plastic ball to do isometric exercises.

*Insight/Action:*

Insight:

Action:

*Affirmation:*

I act as if it is already so, and it is.

## Menu Options
### "Fuel For the Day"

---

**BREAKFAST**

Special K Cereal and Fruit:

1 cup Special K serial (not strawberry), sweetened with

2 teaspoons 100% all fruit jam

1 tablespoon sliced unsalted almonds

½ banana

½ cup skim or low-fat milk

---

*Put all of the above ingredients into a bowl.*

**Snack**

Fruit

---

**LUNCH**

High-Burning Mac N Cheese:

1 cup cooked whole wheat macaroni

½ cup non-fat cottage cheese

3 tablespoons mozzarella cheese from skim milk

1 teaspoon mustard

*Cook macaroni. Top with cottage cheese, mix in mustard to taste, and mozzarella*

---

*Cheese. Add a fruit or vegetable or salad.*

**Snack Boost**

2 dried apricots

2 unsalted almonds

*(in a Zip-loc snack bag)*

---

**DINNER**

Sirloin Steak and Yam:

4 oz. sirloin steak (trimmed and grilled)

4 oz. yam (heated in microwave until soft, sprinkled with cinnamon on top)

1 cup steamed vegetables

---

**Snack**

Chocolate Shake:

3 oz. Westsoy Lite chocolate soy milk

½ banana

*Mix in a blender until tall and frothy.*

*Your day was:* Approximately 1,170 calories, 1,328 mg. sodium, and 117 mg. cholesterol

| 24% protein | 55% carbohydrates | 21% fat |
|---|---|---|

# Week Two

## Responsibility

You will learn to live your life one day at a time. Make each day the best day of your life through positive interaction with yourself. You will choose to be responsible, enjoy your achievements as well as your dreams. You will transform your life through the practice of a working life model. You will learn that your answers are within you. Your inner communication moves you to overcome limitations and inspires you to reach the star quality that you are. Take responsibility for your life today. Respond to it from the inside out.

**Day 8   Accept Personal Responsibility**

**Day 9   Obsessive/Addictive Behavior, What's Your Habit?**

**Day 10   Keep It Simple**

**Day 11   Let Things Unfold**

**Day 12   Acting Out?**

**Day 13   Build Character**

**Day 14   The Formula For Success**

# Day 8

**Part I.**  **Accept Personal Responsibility**

**Part II.**  **Dieting Is A No, No**

**Part III.**  **Know Your Power Plays**

## Just For You (<u>Y</u>our <u>O</u>wn <u>U</u>niqueness)

Write a letter to a special friend, tell him or her how you think of and care for his or her well-being.

# Day 8
## Part I:  Accept Personal Responsibility

Personal responsibility means that you, and you alone, are responsible for what you do. You accept that you are the creator and maintainer of your own world. Few people accept personal responsibility for their lives. Mediocrity and failure can often be traced to lack of a sense of personal responsibility.

People prefer to blame others, institutions, the country, or even the weather, rather than admitting that they are responsible for themselves, how they act, and the results.

While you may not necessarily be responsible for your environment and for the behavior of others, you are responsible for how you have chosen to react. You are responsible for what you are and the way you act.

Until you assume personal responsibility, you will always be caught in a swarm of circumstances that make you feel helpless and futile. When you express personal responsibility, you can move toward those environments that fortify your finer qualities and those individuals who applaud your efforts and encourage your dreams. You will attract them like a magnet.

You were given life. There were guarantees that came with it. These guarantees are the law of life: what you sow, you reap; what you believe, you become; and life is yours to live. But you were also given the freedom to choose your own thoughts and to steer your life in any way you saw fit. Although there are hazards to living, certain risks, there are also ways to make life an exciting adventure. Life has uncertainties, challenges, trials, obstacles, and chances. It is up to you to face the challenges of life, to seize the initiative and plan your future. Work daily at your plan, choose to take responsibility for your life.

# Day 8
## Part II:                    Dieting, It's a No, No

It has been reported across the globe that crash diets are dangerous. Princess Diana led the experts into "Royal Reality" when she wrote about eating disorders and her experience with it. We are aware of the failure of weight loss programs, but the $20 billion dollar business is still alive and well. No fat trimmed here; the image business is larger than life.

Others are saying support groups and behavior modification strategies have been designed to enhance life changes and weight loss. Right now, weight programs use behavior modification for helping people to stick to the diets that the corporation has created. This forced behavior can produce a feeling of deprivation and constant possibility for failure. Weight-loss programs have been revamped but the diet professionals still want to take responsibility for your body, for the profit of the corporation. Attempting to have you use willpower alone can only compound the challenge for most people. Consider will power as direction rather than drive, or push. You don't need will power on a behavior plan that you create. It works for you.

Diets often create a feeling of deprivation for the dieter. You hear "that's a no, no" in your mind. There are many types of diets out there. There is the type that says "Grit your teeth and say no to all the good stuff, eat hard boiled eggs, cottage cheese, carrot and celery sticks." A comedian once said, "No wonder dieters are so mean, they're starved and deranged." Other diets allow all types of "forbidden" pleasures, wine, desserts, bread, and hamburgers. Why do dieters still feel deprived? Unless you have foods of your own choosing, you still feel deprived.

We want to select and choose what we eat and not be forced to eat what someone else chooses. The power of suggestion takes over and whatever we are told we cannot have is what we want. Diets set you up for cheating. The diet can keep you full but not satisfied. Everything seems to be a no, no.

Freedom is the power to choose to eat what you want without guilt. Listen to your inner voice. Your body talks. Do a little communicating with your body and identify all of your own no-no's. They are always unique to you. When you do, you will not want to eat items that do not agree with you and you will live free of food guilt, free to be over weight.

*The Fad Diets are for a day     "For A Day"*

You have seen that changing old habits and attitudes about weight have been a process that develop over time.  Releasing weight does not happen overnight.  Yet, there is an incredible appeal to the promise of a quick weight reduction.  Advertisements for new or "recycled" fad diets continuously appear everywhere.  Remember, the fad diet is for a day.  Here's how to identify a fad diet:

1.     Does it claim a giant weight loss in a short period of time?

2.     Does it focus on *a* specific food or pill that will miraculously "burn up" fat, "keep you feeling full," or suppress appetite?

3.     Does it claim you won't need to exercise and will still lose weight?

4.     Does it require special equipment or expensive specialty foods?

5.     Does it limit personal food choices and require eating at specific times?

*Skipping Meals*

Skipping meals and not eating for hour's sets your body up, you become good at slowing down your metabolism to store calories.  People, who are the weight they want to be, eat when they are hungry and burn the excess during the three to four hours in between.  You want to have a good, fast burning metabolism.  Eating every three to four and one half hours is a good way to insure this.  Being hungry at a time when your body should be hungry is a good sign.  You have taken in the nutrients you need to function at your top energy levels and you have burned what you did not need.  Your body is working on schedule.  It is time to eat again.

Because there are times when you eat out, you will find it necessary to plan your meals.  The point is not to skip meals, it is fattening.  You will learn later how to determine physical hunger versus emotional hunger.  Dieting is a no-no.

# Day 8
## Part III:                    Know Your Power Plays

One of the buzz words that we hear in our communication today is power. This word is frequently used and just as frequently not defined. What do you mean when you say, that it is a powerful person, I have power over this or that, or someone is using their power to control a situation or do not give away your power? Power when defined academically is the ability to do or act, to express strength or force; it is energy and finally it is authority. These qualities make up the description of personal power. Each of us has the ability to do or act, to express strength and energy. Each of us has power.

Authority, one of the key qualities of personal power, is broken down as having authored something or having written or created it. Power, then, is your ability to exercise authority by expressing your creation (your life) with strength and energy. No person or thing can take your power.

Your personal power lies within you. Nothing happens in your life unless it first occurs as an idea or thought within you, you author it. If you desire something, you think of ways to get it. You will recognize the answer when it comes to you. If you can recognize the answer, it has come from something that you have already experienced or have known. Try something new, different. Go outside your "box" (what is familiar). Allow your mind to come up with new ideas, new opportunities. Give them a try. You may be pleasantly surprised at your new-found power. This process of living is acting from your personal power, which always happens from the inside out. While it is a simple experience that happens to you all day every day, you tend to continue to look outside yourself for answers, your happiness, and your personal power.

There are two ways that you can accomplish your goals or meet your personal needs with success. The first is looking outside yourself for the answer, thinking that money, jobs, people or beauty will work it out. You look to people to satisfy your needs, you use a quick fix and magic button way to an easy solution. These outside tactics can band-aid your needs, your hurts, your desires for a time, but you will find yourself quickly looking again for more satisfaction, more things. The second alternative is to use personal power to achieve your goals. To hear the answers from within, feel the motivation and experience the ultimate satisfaction of accomplishment. This is sure and lasting power for you have created it. You've got the power. Try the second alternative by using the following power plays:

## Power Plays (Strategic Actions)

In any game or sport the "plays" are the strategies used to win. You, too, need strategies to use in your life. Here are some suggestions of strategies that can be used to change your weight and win the weight game.

Play 1   Know Your Game

- What are your goals for weight?
- Define your goal clearly. See it, be it.
- Keep it just for you (your own uniqueness). Don't compete, compare, or attempt to be a look-alike!
- Visualize it, own it.
- Write down your goal, not just weight but your total image.

Play 2   Play *Your* Best Game

- Build a belief system (knock out blocks, offenses, interferences, negative setbacks)
- Overcome negative programming--build "word power."
- Establish winning lifestyles, shoot your best shot. Be your best self at all times.
- Develop support from others, keep your environment positive (people, friends, work, and home).

Play 3   Go for the Goal

- Act as if you are the person you want to be: slim, fit, healthy.
- Follow through every day, practice, practice.
- When you miss the target, take a time out and begin again.

It's your game; you are a winner because you played it....!

*Exercise:* (outdoors 30 minutes)

Walk out 15 minutes and back.

**Insight/Action:**

Insight:

Action:

**Affirmation:**

*Even if you are on the right track, you'll get run over if you just sit there.*

# Menu Options

**"Fuel For the Day"**

---

**BREAKFAST**

Peanut Butter and Banana:

2 rice cakes

1 tablespoon Laura Scudder's natural peanut butter

½ banana

½ cup Knudsen's fat-free cottage cheese

½ cup fruit

---

*Spread peanut butter on rice cakes. Place sliced banana on top of peanut butter and rice cakes. Eat cottage cheese and fruit on the side.*

**Snack**

Fruit

---

**LUNCH**

Chicken Pita:

1 whole wheat pita bread

½ cup diced cooked skinless chicken

Lettuce and tomato

1 tablespoon Hidden Valley Light ranch dressing

*Fill pita with chicken, lettuce, tomato and ranch dressing.*

Baby carrots

---

**Snack Boost**

Strawberry Soy Shake

½ cup Westsoy Lite soy milk (vanilla, chocolate or strawberry)

1 cup frozen or fresh strawberries

*Mix ingredients in blender until tall and frothy.*

---

**DINNER**

Bean and Cheese Burrito:

½ cup Rosarita fat-free refried beans

1 tablespoon low-fat shredded cheddar cheese

1 whole wheat tortilla

*Spoon beans into tortilla. Sprinkle cheese on top of beans. Roll up tortilla. Heat in microwave for 2 minutes on high. Have a green salad with five small cooked shrimp and 1 tablespoon fat-free salad dressing*

---

**Snack**

Jam Muffin and Cocoa:

½ whole wheat English muffin

1 teaspoon Smucker's Simply Fruit jam

1 cup of diet cocoa

*Your day was:*   Approximately 1,185 calories, 2,610 mg. sodium, and 87 mg. cholesterol

| 29% protein | 53% carbohydrates | 18% fat |
|---|---|---|

# Day 9

**Part I.**        **Obsessive/Addictive Behavior, What's Your Habit?**

**Part II.**       **Sodium Savvy**

**Part III.**      **It's Personal, Not Public**


**Just For You (<u>Y</u>our <u>O</u>wn <u>U</u>niqueness)**

Go to a public place and people watch, learn from others, and count the people with high energy. What makes them stand out in the crowd? What are their special assets?

# Day 9
## Part I: Obsessive/Addictive Behavior, What's Your Habit?

It is, more often than not, easy to recognize an alcoholic or drug addict. More subtle addictions are those of shopping, work, or eating. Who do you know that does not have some obsessive behavior or bad habit? There are not many people who are free of addiction. This sounds so negative, and yet it is true.

When we look at the alcohol, cigarette or drug addict it is easy and appropriate to see that they are out of balance. They are not in balance with their body design. Health is clearly not present or it is distorted. Memory and habit control our choices relative to our biological make up and behavior. In order for your cells to change, they must be in tune with your blue print or body design. Each cell has intelligence; it is where memories, functions and tendencies are stored. If your blueprint or design is distorted, then a distorted cell will result.

If this is true, you must choose to transform the design in memory, to get rid of the addiction. The addicts are told they will always "own" the addiction and are encouraged to fight it, to will them through a constant vigilance to "kick the habit." Will, as we define it, is direction, a target, not push or force. The addict will give up a habit automatically when offered a greater source of satisfaction. That satisfaction can be learning to love yourself through discipline and personal direction. You will no longer be obsessed about filling an empty void in your life with anything outside your body, such as food, but you will fill your life with activities that are healthy and fun. Do not judge how often this happens, the goal is to become conscious of your eating patterns and understand the satisfaction associated with it. Identify new satisfaction, accomplishment, success.

### Alcohol and Weight

Most alcoholics are thin. Why? Alcohol is very high in calories so drinkers feel satisfied and do not want to eat. Because they do not eat regularly, the calories that they drink are burned and are not used to develop muscle.

If you are not an alcoholic, but a social drinker, when you add alcohol to your diet, you are adding calories that in most cases are not counted. The alcohol also makes you relaxed and not alert to how much you are eating, hence you eat more. The drinks are usually accompanied by snacks such as chips, dip, salsa and so forth. These snacks are also high in calories. The result is double the calories, double the weight. Consider ordering tea or coffee before your meal instead of an alcoholic beverage. The people, the environment and the mood are the same. They are the purpose for the event. Do not depend on the alcohol to make the event a success; you are fooling yourself in most cases if you do.

Overcome food addiction:

You may want to use the following:

- The New Transformation Model presented in week one
- Meditation
- Exercise
- Cleansing the body
- Lots of "Just For You" exercises, make up your own

Add this five-step process to your ideas of overcoming addictive behavior in eating:

1. When you find yourself eating something your centered self has suggested you not eat, ask yourself if you really want this food item. Why? (Motive) Is your desire based upon hunger or emotion?

2. If you must eat, put it on a plate, set the table, get a napkin and utensils even if you do not need them, use them anyway. Do it alone so you will have no distractions, no music, and no radio. Yes, put those chips on a plate!

3. As you are eating, pay attention to your body. Feel the food digest, feel the taste in your mouth, smell it, savor it. Does it satisfy your immediate need?

4. Take out a piece of paper or small journal book and immediately record what you felt at the time you ate and what you ate. Keep a record of the items you eat out of the eating rhythm, whether it was conscious or automatic. What sub-personality was in charge? Was it hunger? If you don't want to keep a journal, simply mark a calendar with a sticker on the times you eat out of order.

5. When you avoid the behavior, reward yourself, you deserve it! When something good follows a certain behavior, you tend to repeat that behavior more often. Some people believe that the inherent rewards should be sufficient motivation for making health behavior changes. For example, the inherent

rewards you will receive from taking daily walks may include losing weight, improving your cardiovascular system, and handling stress more effectively. But for many people, these known benefits are not enough; they find that extra rewards can be greater motivators that assist in sustaining the activity.

Learning to give yourself rewards is a large part of behavior management. It demonstrates that you are worthy of treating yourself well and being rewarded for it. Determining what type of reward you deserve is based on the behavior achieved. Rewards must be meaningful to you and are not necessarily items you purchase. Sometimes rewards may take the shape of allocated time to spend with close friends or alone time. They may be special afternoons set aside for hiking or outings.

### Possible Rewards

| | | |
|---|---|---|
| Go to a special movie | Go walk on the beach | Go to a park |
| Attend a symphony | Have a facial | Take a drive |
| Go out to dinner | Enroll in a class | Get a massage |
| Enter a 3K run | Go to the arboretum | Get a manicure |
| Call someone you love | Buy a CD or record | Go on a hike |
| Get a new haircut | Buy some new stationery | Visit a friend |
| Take a hot, luxurious bath | Hire a maid to clean the house | go shopping |
| By plants for a garden | Buy exercise shoes | Dine out |
| Buy a relaxation tape | Time with your children | Personal time |

# Day 9
# Part II:                          Sodium Savvy

You feel you have had a big loss of weight. You say to yourself, "Oh, that's just water weight." Just water weight! Most of your body is made up of water and that can affect your weight evaluation. Therefore, it is a good idea to learn about the water in your body and how to keep it balanced.

Sodium or salt is an essential ingredient in your diet but can cause problems creating excess water, liver ailments, poor kidney functions and hormonal imbalances. It is important to maintain the right amount of salt in your food intake, by eating foods that have natural sodium, and cutting high sodium foods down or eliminating them from your diet.

When you have a diet that is high in salt, you can have a four to six pound gain in one day. Our tissues swim in a salty sea. Salt is the regulator or the maintainer of water in our system, and dissolves substances outside our cells. Sodium holds or retains the water in our tissues, causing the bloating and puffiness we feel. For example, sprinkle salt on a lettuce leaf and watch it wilt. Salt acts as a sponge. Water retention not only causes weight gain but hypertension, headaches, back problems and swollen ankles/hands, as well. Okay, let's just stop shaking...need some suggestions?

## No More Shaking

1.  Use lemon, vinegar, cooking wine, onions, peppers, garlic to enhance the taste of foods.

2.  Eat more fresh and frozen vegetables.

3.  Use high-sodium sauces and condiments sparingly, e.g., soy sauce, steak sauce, mustard, catsup, and relish.

4.  Remove the salt shaker from the table.

5.  Modify recipes to reduce or eliminate the suggested amount of salt.

6.  Avoid foods that are cured and processed:
    • Canned soups
    • salty snack items, e.g., potato chips, crackers, pretzels
    • bacon, ham, luncheon and deli meats

*Consider these foods when reducing sodium intake:*

| Food | Amount | Sodium |
|---|---|---|
| American cheese | 1 oz. | 406 mg. |
| Heinz barbecue sauce | 1 tbsp. | 230 mg. |
| Oscar Meyer bologna | 1 oz. | 241 mg. |
| Kellogg's corn flakes | 1 oz. | 351 mg. |
| Kosher dill pickle | 1 medium | 928 mg. |
| Good Seasons Italian dressing | 1 tbsp. | 198 mg. |
| McDonald's ¼ lb. w/ cheese | 1 | 1,220 mg. |
| Jello chocolate flavored pudding | ½ cup | 514 mg. |
| Pillsbury canned peas | ½ cup | 367 mg. |
| Banquet fried chicken dinner | 11 oz. meal | 1,831 mg. |

*Source: Bowes and Church's Food Values of Portions Commonly Used. J B. Lippincott Co., Philadelphia, 1989.*

# Day 9
## Part III:          **It's Personal, Not Public**

This experience is just for you. When you tell others about what you are doing, many times you will find yourself under criticism, judgement or other negative energy. Many of your loved ones and associates want to be supportive. While you appreciate the love that they express, your answers come from you. Also, it is a personal program; no one can help you do it. All of your successes are your own. You build your life independently. Co-dependence has never been a constructive activity. Self-confidence is built through personal power. It can be learned through this daily activity, if practiced daily. Do not willingly put yourself under public scrutiny. You have nothing to prove. Your results will speak loud and clear. Your life is personal, not public.

*Exercise:*  (outdoors 30 minutes)

Park It Here:  Go to a park.  Swing, hang, twist (on jungle gym), slide, run, skip, be a kid again.

**Insight/Action:**

Insight:

Action:

**Affirmation:**

*Wether life is seen as an opportunity or a butden depenes one one's point of view, not on one's cirmumstances.*

# Menu Options
## "Fuel For the Day"

---

**BREAKFAST**

Vegetable Omelette:

| | |
|---|---|
| ½ cup Eggbeaters | 1/8 cup sliced mushrooms |
| 1/8 cup diced onions | 1 whole wheat toast |
| 2 teaspoons Smucker's Simply Fruit jam | |

---

*Cook mushrooms and onions in a nonstick fry pan sprayed with vegetable oil until soft. Add Eggbeaters and cook until done. Enjoy with toast covered with jam and a fruit on the side.*

**Snack**

Fruit

---

**LUNCH**

Cheese Shrimp Pizza:

1 whole wheat pita topped with

¼ cup meatless spaghetti sauce

2 tablespoons shredded mozzarella cheese made with skim milk

5 medium shrimp

1/8 cup diced green or red peppers

Sliced tomatoes

---

*Cover pita with spaghetti sauce, shrimp, green or red pepper and cheese. Place in toaster oven until brown. Add sliced tomatoes. Enjoy with a salad.*

**Snack Boost**

Celery with Peanut Butter:

2 stalks of celery, each stalk filled with 2 teaspoons Laura Scudder's unsalted natural peanut butter

---

**DINNER**

Broccoli Tuna Melt

3 oz. of tuna packed in water

1 whole wheat English muffin

1 tablespoon shredded cheddar cheese

½ cup cooked broccoli

*Split muffin down middle and warm in toaster oven lightly. Top with tuna (drained) and cover with cheese. Toast until brown and bubbly. Have fruit on the side.*

---

**Snack**

1 cup whole corn puffs (El Molino or Pure & Simple)

1 tablespoon sliced raw unsalted almonds.

*Shake in a bag and enjoy.*

**Your day was:** Approximately 1,274 calories, 2,338 mg. sodium, and 38 mg. cholesterol

| | | |
|---|---|---|
| 27% protein | 53% carbohydrates | 20% fat |

# Day 10

**Part I:**        **Keep It Simple**

**Part II:**       **Water Is Liquid Gold**

**Part III:**      **Communication:**
                            **Tell It Like It Is**

**Just For You (Your Own Uniqueness)**
Go for a walk in a mall or shopping center, get ideas and inspirations
about your new wardrobe, have fun, dream big.

# Day 10
## Part I:                    Keep It Simple

Without simplicity, you experience personal conflicts. You create invisible enemies to fight. In trying to sort out the world, in attempting to have it fit your mindset, you wear yourself out. There is much emotion in the scheme of things, and when you internalize emotion, you over-saturate yourself negatively with script/drama. The result is fatigue and despair.

The whole purpose of your actions is to improve your life. Your goal is to just be. This is where there is a need for simplicity, for letting things go that do not enrich you. Most of your battles are self-created. Often, you whip yourself into frenzy because things fall well below your expectations. Your expectations are usually founded on comparison and competition. *I want what he/she/they have. They have that, I want that.* You think that if you pound long enough and hard enough, you will work things out and you will be satisfied. Will never creates without the balance of love. Balancing will and love is the way of getting things done. Push and drive are not will. Will is direction, it is energy. Push and drive emphasize the power as being outside and drives away the positive. Be simple, be gentle, be patient.

Power is energy, not force. Energy works all the time. It is in harmony with itself. Power is steady, consistent energy, not mere push or force. Let go, flow with life, keep it simple.

# Day 10
## Part II:                 Water Is Liquid Gold

Your very life depends on liquid gold called water. Your body is two-thirds water, or liquid. In order for you to express perfect health, you must keep the life channels open for intelligent action to flow. Water is used by the body to create this liquid. The life liquid in your body contains fresh oxygen, nutrients, antibodies, carbon, hydrogen and more. This intelligent action carries the very cells that move through your body, designated to act by your DNA, or unique blue print. The action of this liquid knows how to be hair, a sweat gland, a heartbeat or a neuron. It is carried through your body by a magic liquid gold that begins as water. Water sustains and replaces the liquid in your body.

It takes about sixty seconds for an oxygen atom, for instance, to make a complete circuit in your body through the blood stream. This blood stream is the river of your body and must be replenished with water.

Water acts like magic in its benefits, as well. It clears skin, makes hair grow and shine, makes your eyes clear, reduces swelling, and is refreshing and satisfying. Further, it makes elimination possible through the kidneys, bowels, breath and skin. Still another benefit is weight reduction and/or maintenance. It is a _must_ for _weight balance_ as it _moves fat_ molecules out of the system through the digestive tract and is eliminated, rather than stagnated, to gather as cellulite under the skin. Cellulite is fat swimming in a body of water holding toxins and poisons. Needless to say, you will not last anyway without water. No more needs to be said; just in case you didn't get it:

> Drink water and you will live beautifully with an ideal body shape. Water is truly the key to weight management. Drinking water is no longer a well-kept secret; you know now, water is liquid gold.

# Day 10
## Part III:           Communication: "Tell It Like It Is."

Even as you continue to make wiser food choices and other health-enhancing lifestyle changes, you may find yourself in social situations where you feel pressure to eat. Planning your response to these situations ahead of time will keep you in control on your way to reaching your weight-loss goal.

High-pressure situations to eat may come from relatives, friends, co-workers, or even strangers. Usually, these people mean well, but it is important for you to use your new assertion skills to politely refuse their gestures when you would really rather not accept the food offered.

In the left column, list difficult scenarios in which you may experience difficulty saying no to offered food. Include in your description who is pressuring you to eat, what that person may be saying, e.g., "Go ahead, one slice won't hurt you" or "I made this just for you." In the right-hand column, write your plan of action. Write out what you might say the next time you are confronted with the pressure to eat.

| Situation | Your Plan of Action |
|-----------|---------------------|
|           |                     |

## The Saboteurs

| Name | When | What to Do | Positive Affirmation |
|------|------|-----------|---------------------|
| **Indulger** "Go ahead, you deserve it!" | • Special occasions. • You lose weight slowly. • When with friends and relatives. | • Splurge on non-food rewards. • Politely say no. Keep food out of sight. • Compensate. | |
| **Perfectionist** "You blew it." "You're not losing enough." "Everyone else can do it, you're lazy." | • You lose slowly. • You splurge. • Comparing with others. | • Work on improving, not perfection. • Plan a splurge allowance. • Splurge small. | |

| Name | When | What to Do | Positive Affirmation |
|---|---|---|---|
| **Victim**<br>"I couldn't help myself"<br>"They made me do it."<br>"Everyone in my family is fat." | • Social occasions.<br>• Illness.<br>• Comparison, competition.<br>• Depression. | • Others can influence you, but you can choose.<br>• Be assertive.<br>• Make your decisions your own.<br>• Do more for yourself. | |
| **Rebel**<br>"What the heck."<br>"I deserve this."<br>"I'll show them." | • When you expect too much. | • Make your eating plan work, avoid binging.<br>• Get out your reward list, use it.<br>• Love yourself. | |

*Exercise:* (outdoors 30 minutes)

Mall Haul:  Go to the mall with morning joggers, walk for 30 minutes.

*Insight/Action:*

Insight:

Action:

*Affirmation:*

*What you want to become is inside of you, stop looking for it outside.*

# Menu Options
## "Fuel For the Day"

**BREAKFAST**
Cheesy Fruity Danish:
2 tablespoons Knudsen's non-fat cottage cheese
1 tablespoon non-fat mozzarella cheese, shredded
1 tablespoon ricotta cheese made from skim milk
2 teaspoons 100% fruit jam (no sugar added)
¼ cup sliced apples, grapes, blueberries or strawberries
1 whole wheat English muffin

*Top split English muffin with cottage cheese and fruit and top with shredded mozzarella cheese. Place in the broiler oven until brown and bubbly.*
**Snack Boost**
Fruit

**LUNCH**
Chicken Pasta Salad:

| | |
|---|---|
| 1 cup cooked whole wheat macaroni | ½ cup cooked diced chicken |
| 1 tablespoon fat-free mayonnaise | ½ cup grapes |
| 2 tablespoons diced celery | 2 tablespoons diced green onions |
| 2 tablespoons diced tomatoes | Mrs. Dash seasoning |

*Mix all of the above ingredients in a bowl and enjoy.*
**Snack**
Strawberry Soy Shake
½ cup Westsoy Lite soy milk (vanilla, chocolate or strawberry)
1 cup frozen or fresh strawberries
*Mix ingredients in blender until tall and frothy.*

**DINNER**
Turkey Burger
3 oz. ground turkey patty
Mrs. Dash seasoning
Lettuce and tomato
1 whole wheat hamburger bun
*Fry turkey patty in a nonstick pan sprayed with vegetable spray. Place between a bun with lettuce, tomato and mustard. Eat with cole slaw.*
*Cole Slaw: ½ cup shredded cabbage mixed with 1 tablespoon fat-free mayonnaise and mustard (to taste)*
**Snack**
Celery with Peanut Butter:
2 stalks of celery, each stalk filled with 4 teaspoons Laura Scudder's unsalted natural peanut butter

*Your day was:*     Approximately 1,198 calories, 1,867 mg. sodium, and 141 mg. cholesterol
                        25% protein               55% carbohydrates              20% fat

# Day 11

**Part I:**         **Let Things Unfold**

**Part II:**        **Calories, Calories: Who's Counting?**

**Part III:**      **Personal Carriage**

## Just For You (<u>Y</u>our <u>O</u>wn <u>U</u>niqueness)

Take a long bubble bath, put on your favorite music, and luxuriate.

# Day 11
## Part I:                   Let Things Unfold

In our fast-paced world, we fail to grasp the simple fact that things unfold in the fullness of time. We want instant results. We want to think as fast as our computers, to move as fast as our cars, to produce as fast as our machines. In the end, in trying to compete with automation, we lose the "center" of our own gravity and fly in a thousand directions. Then we wonder why our lives do not work. We must give ourselves a chance!

The best way to reach your ideal is to set yourself on the path, and allow the process to unfold in the fullness of time. Any over-determined and forceful behavior burns out soon. In trying to grasp too much in one go, you end up grasping too little. Personal will must be measured out and used with discretion. All unfolding processes are delicate, and you must not, in your eagerness, break the thing you love, yourself.

While the world is faster, you yourself are not. In trying to keep up with the whirl of circumstances, you exhaust yourself. What you gain in quantity, you more than lose in quality. It is better to "do a single thing with excellence and have the world beat a path to your doorstep," than to do many things to get by, without much skill and inner direction. In trying to be fast, you miss using your true talents.

What works for automatia does not work for humans. Your process is slower, but fuller, programmed by centuries of evolution. You are slow to learn and slow to master things, but, once you learn and master, your proficiency is marvelous to behold. Walk through life; touch/savor every whit of it to the fullest. The birds are singing just for you, flowers are blooming just for you. Today is life's magnificent gift to you. Open it slowly, enjoy the process.

# Day 11
## Part II:     Calories, Calories, Who's Counting?

Every food item gives you fuel or energy which is measured in units called calories. Your personal needs depend on your own body image. If your weight is correct (correct for you), you know you are getting the right number of calories. If you need to lose or gain weight, you need to pay attention to the fuel (calorie) value of the meals that you eat. There are some foods that supply many calories and some which supply few. No food can be said to be "fattening." It is a total of daily intake that counts toward weight gain or loss. For instance, if you eat one teaspoon of double chocolate cake, it will not affect your total intake drastically, but eat three slices and see the difference.

If you eat more calories than your body requires, you will store the extra calories as fat. Cut back on the calories and fat seems to melt away. It is that simple. Do not put your attention on the things you do not want to experience, such as counting calories. You do not have to count calories. Practice eating healthy foods in smaller portions. Count your blessings, not your calories, and you will see your image change.

The Dietary Guidelines for Americans are based upon seven basic principles for developing and maintaining a healthier diet. They emphasize balance, variety, and moderation.

1. **Eat a variety of foods.**
   To assure yourself an adequate diet of essential nutrients, eat a variety of foods daily from each of the following food groups: fruits, vegetables, whole grains, legumes (dry beans and peas), dairy products, protein (meat, poultry, fish and eggs).

2. **Maintain a healthy weight.**
   Tips for managing your weight:
   - Increase physical activity.
   - Eat less fat and fatty foods. (Keep the omega fats.)
   - Eat less sugar and sweets.
   - Focus on eating fruits, vegetables, whole grains, legumes, low-fat dairy products, and lean meats.
   - Control portion sizes.

3. **Choose a diet low in fat, saturated fat, and cholesterol**.
   Tips for reducing dietary fat and cholesterol:
   - Choose lean cuts of beef, poultry, and fish. Trim excess fat.
   - Eat eggs and organ meats only in moderation.
   - Limit intake of butter, cream, hydrogenated margarines, shortenings, and coconut oil, and foods made from such products.
   - Broil, bake, or boil rather than fry.
   - Read labels carefully to determine amount and type of fat.

4. **Choose a diet with plenty of vegetables, fruits and grain products.**
To increase complex carbohydrates and fiber, select foods such as whole grains, fresh vegetables, and fresh fruits with skins, beans, and peas.

5. **Use sugars only in moderation.**
Tips for decreasing sugar:
- Use less of all sugars including white sugar, brown sugar, raw sugar, honey, and syrups.
- Reduce sugar in recipes by half.
- Eat less food containing sugar.
- Select fresh fruit or fruits canned in their own juice.
- Read food labels carefully. Avoid words ending in "ose."

6. **Use sodium only in moderation.**
Tips to decrease salt intake:
- Read labels carefully, especially on canned, frozen, prepared and convenience foods.
- Cook with herbs and spices instead of salt.
- Cut down on the salt used at the table.
- Limit intake of salty foods such as potato chips, crackers, nuts, popcorn, condiments, pickled foods, cheese, canned items, and cured meats.

7. **If you drink alcoholic beverages, do so in moderation.**
Alcoholic beverages are high in calories and low in nutrients. Moderation is one drink, which may be one bottle (12 oz.) of beer, one glass (4 oz.) of wine or one cocktail (1½ oz.) of distilled spirits.

In the past, claims were not strictly defined. Presently, these claims can only be used if a food meets government definitions. Here are some of the meanings.

| **Label Claim** | **Definition** (per serving of food) |
|---|---|
| Calorie Free | Less than 5 calories |
| Low Calorie | 40 calories or less |
| Light or Lite | 1/3 fewer calories or 50% less fat; if more than half the calories are from fat, fat content must be reduced by 50% or more |
| Fat Free | Less than 1/2 gram fat |
| Low Fat | 3 grams of fat or less |

| Cholesterol Free | Less than 2 mgs. Cholesterol and 2 grams or less saturated fat |
| Low Cholesterol | 20 mgs. Or less cholesterol and 2 grams or less saturated fat |
| Sodium Free | Less than 5 mgs. sodium |
| Very Low Sodium | 35 mgs. or less sodium |
| Low Sodium | 140 mgs. or less sodium |
| Light in Sodium | 50% less sodium |
| High Fiber | 5 grams or more fiber |

This introduction to nutrition facts can heighten your awareness and become a tool that can help you make healthy eating choices.

# Day 11
# Part III:                    Personal Carriage

We appreciate a gift most when it has been carefully and lovingly packaged. Our goal today is to help you develop a sense of style, balance, and physical presentation that adds to your beautiful image.

Personal carriage is the way you sit, stand, walk, and move; it is your nonverbal communication. When you stand tall and carry yourself properly, your body looks better, your clothes fit better, and you appear more alert and dynamic. Good looks and feeling good about yourself depend upon posture, upon keeping your look smooth and fluid.

When sitting, standing, and walking, your body should be in a continuous line.

Take a stand on posture. A person with great posture and fluid, assertive motion is often more attractive than a person with striking features who does not have good posture and moves without assurance.

When you improve your posture, you improve your health. Your body operates most efficiently with correct posture. Digestive troubles, backaches, poor circulation and just plain weariness can be traced to abuse of posture. When certain muscles are stretched unduly and others are weak from neglect, your figure grows slack and your abdomen protrudes, your hips broaden, your midriff bulges and your shoulders slump.

**Your posture shows how you feel about yourself.  Do not sell yourself short.**

You can be positively expressive by keeping your hands quiet.  Sit relaxed, with spine erect and lines moving in one direction.  Practice smooth, continuous, slow motion for a poised appearance that expresses energy in grace.  You should move with an assurance that demands respect.

The posture you choose today affects not only your present appearance, but also determines your health and the shape of your figure for the future.

*Exercise:*  (outdoors 30 minutes)

Park It Here:  Go to local park, swing, hang, and twist on jungle gym, slide--run play.

*Insight/Action:*

Insight:

Action:

*Affirmation:*

Stand for something or you will fall for everything.

# Menu Options
## "Fuel For the Day"

**BREAKFAST**

Hot Apple Oatmeal:

| | |
|---|---|
| 1 cup cooked plain oatmeal | 2 teaspoons 100% all fruit jam |
| ½ cup skim or low-fat milk | ½ cup diced apple |
| ½ teaspoon cinnamon | |

*Cut up apple and cook in microwave until soft and warm. Heat up oatmeal and put in jam to sweeten. Top oatmeal with cooked apples, cinnamon and milk.*

**Snack Boost**

2 dried apricots

3 unsalted almonds

*(In a Zip-loc snack bag)*

**LUNCH**

Soup and Sandwich:

1 can Anderson's fat-free split pea soup

2 tablespoons water

1 slice of pumpernickel bread

2 tablespoons ricotta cheese made with skim milk

1 slice tomato

Black pepper

*Put in a large mug, split pea soup and water. Stir and heat in a microwave until hot. Toast pumpernickel bread and spread ricotta cheese on top. Place tomato on top of cheese and add pepper to taste.*

**Snack**

Fruit

**DINNER**

Spaghetti and Meat Sauce:

¾ cup whole wheat pasta

¼ cup cooked ground turkey

¼ cup spaghetti sauce (Classico or Bertolli) without meat

*Cook pasta in a sauce pan. Drain and top with heated spaghetti sauce and cooked ground turkey. Green salad with 1 tablespoon low-fat salad dressing.*

**Snack**

Frozen Grapes

2 cups grapes

*Rinse grapes until clean. Place in a freezer bag in the freezer overnight.*

***Your day was:*** Approximately 1,182 calories, 1,300 mg. sodium, 131 mg. cholesterol

22% protein       56% carbohydrates       22% fat

# Day 12

**Part I:**       **Acting Out?**

**Part II:**      **Fatty, Fatty, Do Not Take It Personally**

**Part III:**     **Managing Energy Responsibly**

## Just For You (<u>Y</u>our <u>O</u>wn <u>U</u>niqueness)

Dress up and go out to a meal.  Feel beautiful and successful, feel great about yourself.

# Day 12
## Part I:                             Acting Out?

People who have a great degree of "internal control" are ones who feel that they largely determine their destinies by the inner characteristics, attitudes, and resources they develop during their lifetimes. They are identified as "inner-directed" individuals.

People who are externally controlled are those who react and are governed by their environment, institutions, organizations, people, circumstances, and situations in which they happen to find themselves. They relate to life largely by "going along with it." They are known as "outer-directed" people.

Determine your degree of inner and outer direction by answering these questions:

1.    In what ways would the inner-directed person be different from the outer-directed person in the following situations?

    a. Communicate with others, being assertive or permissive.
    b. Attitude toward self-management and making life changes.
    c. Ability to change one's personality, attitudes or habits of behavior.

2.    Do you associate the terms inner- and outer-directed with such terms as introvert and extrovert or positive and negative? In what ways could it be undesirable to put such labels on people?

3.    In what ways could being inner-directed be helpful to you? In what ways could being outer-directed be helpful to you?

4.    Did you have the feeling there was a right or wrong way to answer these questions? If so, why? What effect would the way you are raised, your social and economic background have on your inner- and outer-directed responses to problems or change?

5.    The purpose of this questionnaire is not to establish the attitudes a person should or should not have but simply to help you become aware of the way you respond to life's challenges.

# Day 12
## Part II:
## Fatty, Fatty,
## Do Not Take It Personally

Fat: You cannot take it personally. Most Americans consume a high-fat diet, often as high as sixty percent total fat. Fat, salt and sugar are the ingredients that make the food taste good, or at least that is how most of us are programmed. Variety in tastes is truly found in fresh fruits and vegetables but our taste buds tell us to add fat. You may have thought to yourself from time to time, "I really don't eat that much, I wonder why I maintain these extra pounds?" Take another look at what you are eating and when you are eating it. Fats, salts and sugar are not easy to digest; they just sit on your body. They are stored in places we won't discuss. Don't take fat personally; learn to be aware of the percentages of fat from the foods you eat. Fat intake from calories should be no more than 30 percent per day. Let's look at a few fat facts.

1.  **What is fat?**
    Fat is a more concentrated source of energy than carbohydrate or protein. All fats contain 9 calories per gram, while carbohydrates and protein each contain 4 calories per gram. One teaspoon of fat contains 45 calories.

2.  **What are saturated fats?**
    Saturated fats are usually of animal origin and are usually solid at room temperature. Examples include butter, cream, whole milk and cheese. Among the few vegetable fats that are saturated are coconut oil, palm oil, palm kernel oil (often used in non-dairy cream substitutes, frozen desserts, and many processed foods) and cocoa butter, which is the fat found in chocolate. Saturated fats tend to increase the amount of cholesterol carried in the blood system.

3.  **What are unsaturated fats?**
    These are fats of plant and fish origin and are liquid at room temperature. Vegetable oils vary in their degree of unsaturation. For example, safflower oil, a polyunsaturated fat, is more unsaturated than olive oil, a monounsaturated fat. Omega-3 fatty acids are found in fish, especially salmon, mackerel, tuna and sardines. Recent evidence shows that both types of unsaturated fats, monounsaturates and polyunsaturates, help to lower the amount of cholesterol in the blood *when substituted for saturated fats*.

Remember to always listen to the Boss for direction and guidance about what you eat.

Also, here are a few ideas that may help:

**1. Reduce your meat intake.**
Eat only the leanest cuts and then cut your portion in half. Each serving should be no larger than the palm of your hand. A ten-ounce serving of steak with rice, string beans, and undressed salad amounts to almost 800 calories, 34 percent from fat. Reduce the meat portion to three ounces, stir fry the meat with green beans, you have 424 calories, and the fat drops to 23 percent.

**2. Add more grains, vegetables, fruits and pasta to your meals.**
It is not these foods that have fat; it is the dressing, sour cream and butter that escalate the fat count.

**3. Choose low-fat dairy products.**
Using non-fat or milk with only one or two percent milk fat can bring down the fat count drastically. Go easy on the cheese; it has been called orange lard. If you do not believe it is all grease, heat it and see the grease.

**4. Define fat in prepared foods.**
Learn to read the labels. Low fat, light, and "cholesterol free" have a hidden agenda. Lower than what, leaner than what, compared to what? Check the fat grams, the sodium content, etc., and then make a decision. To tell how many fat grams you can reasonably eat in a day, take the rough number of calories you consume daily, drop the last zero and divide by three. When you eat about 1600 calories per day, you are eating 50-55 grams of fat.

**5. Change your menus to light ones.**
According to Dr. William Costelli, director of the Framingham Heart Study, most Americans eat the same recipes week in and week out. Try low-fat substitutes in your meal planning. Use variety, make eating enjoyable. Do not fry, instead, microwave, steam, braise, boil, barbecue, roast, bake, broil, poach, stew or stir fry (in spray coating or one teaspoon of oil). Instead of basting meat in drippings, use fruit juices, sprayed lemon water or desalted broths.

**6. Watch eating out**.
Make it an occasion rather than a habit because you do not feel like cooking. What we think is fast food takes twice as long to get to than steamed or microwaved foods at home. Most of the time, when we eat fast foods we eat it out of the package in front of the TV, or in the car. These activities cause digestive problems and make eating a boring or hidden activity.

**7. Do not deprive yourself.**
Have occasional treats, if high in fat, eat half the amount. You will learn to enjoy healthy treats. You are not celebrating every day, so when you have an occasion to do so, do it guilt free. When the event is over, be in rhythm with your food intake--cut the fat. Do not take it personally.

# Day 12
# Part III:      Managing Energy Responsibly

Closely linked to time management is energy management. The cardinal rule is that you can only do well what you are in the mood to do. Moods are indications of inner rhythms. They should be respected and not ignored. A mood is a gauge of energy. Don't get caught up in a mood that is negative.

A good mood means that you are experiencing "on-time." You have on-time when your energy is up, when you are interested in doing something, when you can perform in a calm and deliberate manner. You can create "on-time."

A bad mood means that you are experiencing "off-time." You have off-time when your energy is down, when you are not interested in something, and when you can perform only in an agitated and forced manner. It is not true that you work better under pressure. Getting something <u>done</u> is not always a measure of excellence. You can create "on-time" or change it.

On-time can be used to create meaningful experiences for yourself and off-time can be used to rest and recuperate, read your energy and act accordingly.

If you work during off-time, you are depleting your energy, reducing your ability to perform. Off-time work cuts into the positive work that would have followed after rest and recuperation. This poor use of energy can result in error, frustration and rapid fatigue.

On-time is for functioning and off-time is for recuperation. You are not wasting time when you rest. Do it guilt free.

You can take responsibility for your life by using your energy wisely.

There may be times when you are off time and you find that you are worrying, concerned about a situation. If you create a busy "monkey mind," jumping all over your head, try using the "quiet mind" exercise. It works!

Here's how:

**The Quiet Mind**

Have you ever heard a song in your head and couldn't stop hearing it? Many times we have trouble focusing on an idea. What about the times when we stay awake worrying or thinking about a situation? These activities of the mind are sometimes called the "mad monkey" mind. The mad monkey swings from one branch to another in constant movement. How can we quiet our minds?

Exercise

1.  Identify the noisy or busy area of your brain by paying attention to where the activity is, physically.

2.  When you locate the area of your head, place your hand over it without touching your head.

3.  Close your eyes. While your hand is still over this area, shift your attention to the opposite side of your brain.

4.  Where you focus the new attention is your quiet mind, stay there and regroup.

5.  If this doesn't work for you the first time, repeat the exercise until it does.

*Exercise:* (outdoors 30 minutes)

Track your time.  Walk around the track at your neighborhood school.

**Insight/Action:**

Insight:

Action:

**Affirmation:**

*Only those who wil risk going too far…can possibly find out how far one can go.*

# Menu Options
## "Fuel For the Day"

---

**BREAKFAST**
Healthy Egg Muffin:
½ cup Eggbeaters
1 tablespoon shredded cheddar cheese
1 sliced beefsteak tomato
1 whole wheat English muffin (split)
Pepper to taste

---

*Cook up Eggbeaters in nonstick pan (sprayed with vegetable spray). Sprinkle cheddar cheese on top of Eggbeaters. Toast English muffin. Top muffin with tomato, Eggbeaters and cheese, and enjoy. Have a fruit on the side.*

**Snack Boost**
2 dried apricots
3 unsalted almonds
*(In a Zip-loc snack bag)*

---

**LUNCH**
Steak Bowl:

| | |
|---|---|
| ½ cup cooked brown rice | 2 tablespoons chopped red bell pepper |
| 3 ounces diced sirloin steak | 2 tablespoons chopped green onions |
| Salsa to taste | 1 tablespoon shredded fat-free cheddar cheese |

*Mix all ingredients in a bowl. Have fruit on the side.*

---

**Snack**
Strawberry Soy Shake
½ cup Westsoy Lite soy milk (vanilla, chocolate or strawberry)
1 cup frozen or fresh strawberries
*Mix ingredients in blender until tall and frothy.*

---

**DINNER**
3 oz. broiled salmon (with lemon and Mrs. Dash)
Yam (cooked in microwave until soft)
Salad with 1 tablespoon non-fat dressing

---

**Snack**
Baked Apple
1 apple
2 teaspoons 100% fruit jam (no sugar)
*Cook apple in microwave until soft. Put jam on top of apple to sweeten.*

*Your day was:*   Approximately 1,185 calories, 719 mg. sodium, 194 mg. cholesterol
   29% protein          48% carbohydrates          23% fat

# Day 13

**Part I:**     **Build a Fine Character**

**Part II:**     **Real Versus Psychological Hunger**

**Part III:**     **Be Positively Coordinated**

## Just For You (<u>Y</u>our <u>O</u>wn <u>U</u>niqueness)

Sit for an hour alone and listen to your favorite music,
practice being quiet. It pays off.

# Day 13
## Part I:  Build A Fine Character

"Your life is what your thoughts make it," said Marcus Aurelius.

If you are inconsiderate, pessimistic, cruel, weak, drab, irritable and undetermined, then your thoughts are of envy, conceit, cynicism, self-pity, suspicion, indecision, criticism and inferiority; and your life is one of worry, tension, despondency, frustration, unhappiness, failure, sickness, poverty, and boredom. Why is it that they say negative experience can build character? As you triumph over such an experience you build character muscle.

If, however, you are enthusiastic, decisive, optimistic, considerate, friendly, curious, sincere and relaxed, then your thoughts are of understanding, anticipation, confidence, patience, and belief; and your life is one of success, recognition, security, energy, achievement, growth, adventure, health and love. You, too, can triumph.

Many years ago, James Allen, in his book, <u>As a Man Thinketh</u>, wrote: "One is literally what he/she thinks, character is the complete sum of our thoughts....A noble and God-like character is not a thing of favor or chance, but is the natural result of continued effort in right thinking, the effect of long cherished association with God-like thought." Today, he would have written as a person thinks. Build a fine character by building constructive positive thoughts. Practice managing your thoughts. You've got the power!


# Day 13
## Part II:  Real Versus Psychological Hunger

Today, you are going to identify your real physiological hunger. If you know your body is really physiologically hungry, then eat. When your body needs fuel, it will tell you with physical symptoms. Listen to your body, it will direct you to the food it needs for fuel. One way to identify real physical hunger is to remember if you have eaten a balanced meal within the past four hours. A balanced meal can contain fruits or vegetables, complex carbohydrates, simple carbohydrates and a moderate amount of protein. When your body is regulated, you will be hungry approximately every four hours. Your body changes chemically every three to four hours. So, even if you ate all the food on a buffet in Las Vegas, your body would still be hungry after that period. You cannot stockpile food.

We have heard of people fasting for forty days, or even starving in a desert for weeks. The reason why we can last under those drastic circumstances is that our bodies adjust, and come with a miraculous healing power. If the human body is not fed for long periods of time, it compensates, the metabolism slows down. Metabolism is the burning of calories to create energy. It exists to fuel the body with a sophisticated energy system. We are always burning calories. Even in our sleep, our bodies burn approximately twelve calories every ten minutes.

When the body thinks it is being starved, it will store the calories as fat in preparation for the next starvation period. Eat when you are physically hungry. Many people eat to satisfy emotional or psychological needs. The clue is when the desire for food comes from outside us. An example, "I'm bored, what can I eat?" Outside food stimulant. Another example, "I feel so sad, I think I'll have something to eat. I'm lonesome; I think I'll have some popcorn." Question the real satisfaction; ask yourself, "Will food solve the problem?" Maybe it is a psychological hunger and can better be served by working out the problem. Food hunger is purely physiological; anything else is not physical hunger. Watch out!! This is how we create lifelong negative food responses.

Don't be fooled by your eye appeal or outside stimuli. Do not eat just because it is 12 p.m. or someone has prepared a meal or snack for you or just because it's in front of you.

### The Food-Feeling Connection

Eating is often more than a physical need for nourishment. Emotional or psychological eating can result from many types of triggers. After years of reaching for food for comfort, this type of eating becomes a learned response, although a negative one, for dealing with unpleasant and difficult situations.

*I have identified the following personal Food-Feeling Connections which I will work on changing:*

The Feeling                              My Current Response

103

Changing your response to food and your Food-Feeling Connections may be the most challenging and most rewarding behavior change that you can make. Some people look toward food as a method to cope with difficult situations or feelings such as stress, boredom, loneliness, and hurt. Food isn't the answer.

Breaking the connections between food and feelings requires an awareness and love for you.

# Day 13
## Part III:       Be Positively Coordinated

Success in life depends upon how you coordinate major life activities. You will find that you can get everything done if you are organized and honest about what you can and cannot do. You are where you are today because of discipline. Develop behavior modification skills that assist you in coordinating the activities of your life in order to be free to enjoy the precious time that you have. Work smarter not harder is a great adage to remember.

Observe yourself as you develop ways to modify or change behavior. Look at yourself, question who and where you are. Remember, whatever you resist, you attract. Know then what you are resisting: define it and let it go. Use the visualization and affirmation exercise.

Coordination and poise create the confidence that is highly desirable. This confidence comes from being acquainted with the many things that stimulate intelligence and personal growth. It is being in the know about what's going on, the news, important people and happenings, past and present, which affect our environment. You develop confidence as you learn bit by bit from what you do, read and observe. Learn about art, music, ballet, great writers and philosophers. Instead of watching three or four hours of television daily, read a novel, learn a language or develop a new skill.

Coordinate your leisure activities. What different places can you visit? Plan to spend your weekend doing something special. Perhaps it can be a sight-seeing trip, maybe a lunch at an interesting restaurant, an evening at the theater, or possibly, just a try at a different sport. Any worthwhile change of place or pace will put more zest in your life.  Make your life full and complete, be positively coordinated.

*Exercise:* (outdoors 30 minutes)

Explore a new territory:  Drive to a new neighborhood within your community.  Walk 15 minutes out, 15 minutes back.

*Insight/Action:*

Insight:

Action:

*Affirmation:*
*The ways you think that you are, not the ways that you really are, are the bars on your personal prison.*

# Menu Options
## "Fuel For the Day"

---

**BREAKFAST**

Peanut Butter and Banana:

2 rice cakes

1 tablespoon Laura Scudder's natural peanut butter

½ banana

½ cup Knudsen's fat-free cottage cheese

½ cup fruit

---

*Spread peanut butter on rice cakes. Place sliced banana on top of peanut butter and rice cakes. Eat cottage cheese and fruit on the side.*

**Snack Boost**

Fruit

---

**LUNCH**

Turkey Waldorf Salad Sandwich:

½ cup diced cooked turkey

1 tablespoon chopped walnuts

¼ cup chopped celery

1 tablespoon fat-free mayonnaise

Lettuce / tomatoes

1 slice of pumpernickel bread (toasted)

*Mix first 7 ingredients in a bowl and place on top of pumpernickel bread.*

---

**Snack**

Veggies and Bean Dip:

½ cup Rosarita fat-free refried beans in microwave

Dip your favorite raw vegetables (mushrooms, broccoli, jicama, etc.

---

**DINNER**

Shrimp Kabob:

5 medium shrimp

1 cubed cooked potato

5 chunks of pineapple (without sugar, packed in its own juice)

5 cherry tomatoes

Mushrooms

*Put above ingredients through a skewer. Marinate in fat-free Italian dressing. Broil until brown, 5-7 minutes.*

---

**Snack**

Blueberry Cream Cheese Parfait:

1 cup blueberries (fresh or frozen)          2 tablespoons Cool Whip Lite

1 tablespoon Philadelphia Light cream cheese  1 teaspoon vanilla

*Fold together all ingredients and serve in a bowl. Makes 1 serving.*

*Your day was:*  Approximately 1,266 calories, 1,961 mg. sodium, and 102 mg. cholesterol

25% protein                60% carbohydrates                15% fat

# Day 14

**Part I:**   **The Formula for Success**

**Part II:**   **Use Food to Your Advantage**

**Part III:**   **Insight and Action**

### Just For You (Your Own Uniqueness)

Rent a movie that inspires you, or just makes you feel good.
Treat yourself to some popcorn, if you'd like.
(My upbeat film is *Forrest Gump*.)

# Day 14
## Part I:                 The Formula for Success

There is a formula that works to bring your goals, visions and dreams to reality. The formula goes like this: First you have the idea, a goal or dream of what you want. Second, you see it, and add visualization. Third, you add the appropriate behavior, the attitude, the action. All of these activities must be topped by belief and practice. This all equals success. Now we must "act as if."..you must practice.

Practice makes perfect. If you "act as if" you have a healthy body or attitude, your computer mind will respond to this behavior, or belief, for your life works on the action of your belief. You must first commit yourself to seeing yourself eating healthy, having a positive attitude. Visualize releasing excess weight, see it melt, see it go through and out, see it leave in a constructive, permanent way and it will. This activity is demonstrated by many athletes and public speakers. As you practice this new behavior, as you "act as if," you strengthen your experience of success. When you practice the desired activity, it will happen naturally, easily and effortlessly, because you have made the blueprint for its success, you have practiced it, and now it is truth. Do this activity and increase self-confidence. All you need to do is "act as if" you have the confidence that you desire. Choose a specific goal that you would like to achieve, commit to it. It works...but you will never know until you try it. Remember:

### The Formula For Success

$$\frac{\text{Idea} + \text{Visualization} + \text{Desired Behavior}}{\text{Belief} + \text{Practice}} = \text{Success}$$

# Day 14
## Part II:        Use Food to Your Advantage

The most difficult aspect of changing eating habits is giving up old patterns. When we eat snacks, we tend to think of it as cheating. Our old pattern is to eat the snacks and feel guilty. Most snacks are not planned. We feel hungry; we are on the run, at a party, or on a work break. What do we do? We respond to this urge by grabbing a candy bar, carbonated drink, chips or cookies. Because they are empty calories and simple carbohydrates, they just do not satisfy you for a long period. The snack break becomes a vicious circle, hunger-guilt-hunger. "Time out!" Go back to the program here; make sure that you have a healthy snack between meals. Yes, it is an important component to have, no guilt involved. What is the "but" in this activity? The "but" is that the snack must be planned. A great snack tucked into your desk drawer, glove compartment, refrigerator, pocket or purse is just right. Enjoy it, feel energized; you are on target. Your menu options give you great snack ideas.

It is time for you to use food to your advantage. One definition of power in the dictionary is the ability to make a choice. There are all kinds of choices, but if we don't have information, we don't know how to make good choices, and we feel powerless. You are going to learn the information that people, who are healthy and slim, and stay that way, already know.

Slim and healthy people do not think of food in the way of calories, solutions to problems or deprivation. They are selective of the food they eat, they eat what they enjoy. They eat when they are hungry until satisfied, not because someone invites them to, or sets food in front of them, or out of fear. Listen to your body; learn to use food to your advantage.

Satisfaction is not only physical and emotional; it is also mental (in your brain).

## Satiety Centers

Certain brain centers control the sensations associated with appetite, hunger and satisfaction. These centers normally encourage people to eat an amount of food that provides the right amount of energy for their needs. *The feeding centers make people want to eat.* You can use this to your advantage. When you want something to eat and know it is not best for you, you can satisfy the brain, trick the feeding centers, by eating it in a smaller portion. Eat the item(s) but eat less and less each time you eat it. The brain and emotions are satisfied and soon the portion gets smaller and smaller until you can eliminate the food item altogether. You have tricked your brain into satisfaction.

The satiety centers act as a break on the feeding centers. They make us feel satisfied and we stop eating. The feeding centers are extremely complicated mechanisms. Their function may be affected by emotional pressures or physical imbalances, diseases, sickness. For example, deep depression, grief, tragedy can cause some people to stop all physical activity, including the desire to eat. Others cannot stop; they run around and eat non-stop. Genes play a part in the function of these satiety centers. Your awareness of the centers can help you to manage your food wisely. Go back, ask your body, is this physiological or psychological hunger? How else can I satisfy my need at this time? Use food to your advantage.

# Day 14
## Part III:                    Insights and Action

Write down all the insights that have come to you as a result of participating so far. What actions have you taken? Personalize them. Outline how you can use them. It is not enough to learn stimulating ideas, you must write and think about them and make them part of your mental awareness, but most of all put them into action, make a commitment to modify your behavior, your life. Repeat this exercise after the 21st day. Do this insight and action exercise.

*Exercise*

Write a personal response to the first 13 days of this experience. What insight have you had? What actions have you taken as a result? This exercise will allow you to evaluate the effectiveness of this experience. It is rather a checkpoint, for you to know if it is for you. Congratulations. Keep moving forward.

Insight:


Action:

*  *  *

*Exercise:*  (outdoors 30 minutes)

Keep it natural!  Take a nature walk.  Go to the beach, park, lake, and river--have fun!

*Insight/Action:*  (you have already done it, but you may want to write about today anyway)

<u>Insight</u>:

<u>Action</u>:

*Affirmation:*

**Enjoy your achievemens as well as your dreams.**

# Menu Options
## "Fuel For the Day"

---

**BREAKFAST**

Cheesy Fruity Danish:

2 tablespoons Knudsen's non-fat cottage cheese
1 tablespoon non-fat mozzarella cheese, shredded
1 tablespoon ricotta cheese made from skim milk
2 teaspoons 100% fruit jam (no sugar added)
¼ cup sliced apples, grapes, blueberries or strawberries
1 whole wheat English muffin

---

*Top split English muffin with cottage cheese and fruit and top with shredded mozzarella cheese. Place in the broiler oven until brown and bubbly.*

**Snack Boost**
2 dried apricots
3 unsalted almonds
*(In a Zip-loc snack bag)*

---

**LUNCH**

Egg Salad Sandwich:

3 hard-boiled egg whites
1 tablespoon fat-free mayonnaise
1 teaspoon mustard
2 tablespoons chopped celery
2 tablespoons chopped red onions
2 slices whole wheat bread

*Mix egg whites and the next 4 ingredients in a bowl. Spread on bread. Eat with a fruit.*

---

**Snack**
Fruit

---

**DINNER**

4-oz. baked chicken breast (skinless)
3 oz. yam (cooked in microwave until soft), sprinkled with cinnamon
Salad with 1 tablespoon of low-fat dressing

---

**Snack**
Jam Muffin and Cocoa:

½ whole wheat English muffin
1 teaspoon Smucker's Simply Fruit jam
1 cup of diet cocoa

*Your day was:*   Approximately 1,135 calories, 2,207 mg. sodium, 85 mg. cholesterol
25% protein               61% carbohydrates               14% fat

# Week Three

## Love

In this last week of the 21-day experience, you will take a long look at yourself, an assessment of your special qualities. You will think of your presence as a gift to the world. You will discover that you are unique, one of a kind. You will know that your life can be what you want it to be through your conscious thought, your choice, your beliefs, but most of all through love.

# Day 15

Part I:        **Self-Acceptance Is Unconditional Love**

Part II:       **Take Stock Of Your Wardrobe**

Part III:     **Create A Unique Environment**

## Just For You (Your Own Uniqueness)

Do something creative, draw a picture, write a poem, take a photo, tell a story, make a kite, whatever suits your fancy— just allow your creative expression to act.  Have fun.

# Day 15
## Part I:  Self-Acceptance Is Unconditional Love

The first step to a life-enhancing attitude is to move beyond all negative images of you.  Put aside the limited person you feel you have become, the person you feel circumstances have molded.  Avoid this reality, create a new one.  What you give your attention to becomes your reality, your experience.  Stop working on your problems, when you practice the problems you get good at them, put your attention on the solutions and the energy that you give to the solution will build, soon you will be living from answers not problems.

Shun your own shortcomings and live as if you were someone exceptional, special, and incredible.  Act like a star.  Your specialness should be the center of your new reality.

Psychologists tell us that children are non-logical, and believe that they are magical and invincible.  But as children grow up, they are "educated" to believe their shortcomings.  This is what passes for logical understanding.

Most of us are raised to believe in what we cannot do.  Rare and exceptional is the person with a mind oriented toward what he or she can do.  The belief in lack is pervasive.  It is time to change this programming and resort to the childlike faith in ourselves and in life that we all once had.  We must be as little children.  This is the best attitude of all, the attitude of deep and unconditional self-acceptance and openness to the wonders of life, enjoying the freedom of the child.

Find within yourself the child who might not have measured up.  Tell that child that everything is well, that the child is free to be itself, that fitting in with the rules of others has not lessened its beauty, magic, or charm.  Accept yourself, love yourself unconditionally.

### Love Yourself Enough to Say No

Why is it so hard to say no?  We live in a world where most people want to be approved, accepted and "good."  Do we take a gigantic risk of losing this approval or status when we say no?  Do you feel that agreement and going along will ensure your acceptance?  We are quick to say to drug addicts, "just say no" but what about the subtler addictions and obsessions?  Can you say no, thank you, if someone prepares food that is not good for you, offers you a meal when it's too late in the evening, insists that you have a piece of cake or other empty calorie dishes because it's a special occasion?

It is difficult to say no when we are in a situation where someone has created something special just for us, out of love. But just as with any other obsessive behavior, if the food, time or situation isn't right, then love yourself enough to say no. The benefits are that you will feel good about caring for yourself and others in your life will love and respect you for standing up for what you believe is right for you.

Love yourself enough to say no.

# Day 15
## Part II:     Take Stock Of Your Wardrobe

Now is the time to sit down with pencil and paper and analyze your life. What activities fill your day? Note every one. Make a list of things you have done in the past month. This list will guide you in choosing clothes that suit your role in life. Looking the part, your image is essential. Now look around you. What are your peers and colleagues wearing? You will want to reflect the image of your lifestyle. While fashion changes, certain styles remain. Be aware of what is in fashion. Read fashion magazines, watch TV fashion shows. Be savvy!

*Exercise*

List your daily activities and evaluate the type of clothing that you need. For example, you will not want to have a predominate wardrobe of casual clothing if your daily activities call for business attire. Have a few pieces of clothing for the special occasions in your life, of course, but the focus of your wardrobe should be in keeping with your lifestyle day to day.

Take stock, do you need to replace or add items? Maybe you should network with a friend by exchanging clothing or go to a vintage thrift shop, where money is no object. Be creative and have fun. Keep your wardrobe simple, it is not true that you do not have a thing to wear. Most of us are looking in our closet for a particular motive in our dressing. If you know the motive you can capitalize on the event with your image. An example of a motive in dressing is, "If I wear this I know I will look like I mean business." It is how we communicate our goals, it is how we create an environment. Understand what the motive is and dress to enhance the situation. Be committed to be your best self. Every one in your environment will respond positively to your best self, if not, it is their experience, not yours. Always look like you mean business. What does wardrobe and dressing have to do with weight management? Create a total image for confidence that will encourage you to look your personal best at all times. Transform your image, transform your life.

### Good Looks and Grooming Tell The Inside Story

Neat and clean are the key words for the well-groomed look. All grooming should be done in private. You should be neat, clean and well organized at all times. Grooming is as important when wearing shorts as it is when wearing formal clothes. It takes planning to appear your best. Have adequate supplies available. Organize all of your supplies in groups, such as skin care supplies, hair supplies, etc. Discard all articles not in use to keep from developing clutter. You are most confident when you are well groomed. Watch for those trouble spots: elbows, knees, heels and knuckles. Work for "neat feet."

Remember that ready-to-wear is a term that should apply to everything you own. Every appearance is your most important one. So, how does wardrobe apply to weight? Looking good encourages you to keep on looking good.

### Plan Your Shopping

Try to become acquainted with the characteristics of good clothes. Examine the clothes in the window or on display in better stores. Observe factors that warrant the expensive price. One who is familiar with the look of quality will be better at shopping, and save money in the long run.

Before buying a garment, check the fit, look over the shoulder seams, darts, length and overall finish (hems, lining, buttons, and zippers).

Know what you want before shopping. Have a plan and shop your plan. Getting a "good buy" can be a matter of luck, but more often it is a matter of careful deliberation. Persons who are always well dressed, who forever find little bargains, have shopping down to a system. They know where to buy and when to buy. They know the sales people in the stores who call when something is in that suits them, or when something is on sale.

When shopping remember that what you buy must do something for you and at the same time enhance your wardrobe. Too often people buy because an article is on sale, and it was a bargain that was hard to pass up. But you must learn to pass up some to keep your closet and mind clear. In any case, most of these bargains end up as expensive when they hang in the closet, waiting for the right time. Still, there are indeed bargains. You can expand your wardrobe budget considerably and get as much as 25 percent to 35 percent more value for your clothing dollar when you shop wisely.

### *Measure Your Own Fashion Proportions*

1. Perfect body ratio is four equal parts: Top of head to chest, chest to hip, hip to knee, knee to heel. You can compensate for unequal ratios in your body through your wardrobe. For example, if your waist is short, wear longer jackets.

2. Measure chest, waist, hips, arms and legs. Where are you longer or larger? Do you have thin legs, heavy legs, knock-knees, and so forth.

3. Covering or hiding areas is not always the answer. Large, loose fitting clothing has a tendency to make you appear larger. Layers are very effective when made of coordinated materials or flowing lines. Ask your store professional or wardrobe consultant for assistance. Follow your mind, ask the "Boss."

# Day 15
# Part III:     Create A Unique Environment

Who you are is expressed in your environment, the one that you create around you. Where you live is always where you are right now; so your environment is your body, your aroma, your colors, your home, where you work, walk and live.

Your body design dictates the type of environment where you are most comfortable. Refer back to your body design. Note the temperature, season, color, and aroma and pace that is best for you. Do it, or you allow yourself to live in a toxic environment that throws you off balance and triggers ill health and weight imbalance.

Where you live is very important in your life for it tells again a story about what you think of yourself, how orderly you are and what your organizational skills are. It would probably be alright if you only knew, but your environment tells the world what you think of yourself. Be sure your message is what you want it to be.

.

*Exercise:* (indoors 30 minutes)

Help from pros: Yoga on television.

*Insight/Action:*

Insight:

Action:

*Affirmation: Be Present....*
*I might as well enjoy here while I'm here, cause there aint no here there.*

# Menu Options
## "Fuel For the Day"

---

**BREAKFAST**
1 cup Special K cereal (not strawberry)
2 teaspoons 100% all fruit jam
1 tablespoon sliced unsalted almonds
½ banana

---

½ cup skim or low-fat milk          *Put all ingredients in a bowl.*
**Snack Boost**
2 dried apricots
3 unsalted almonds
*(in a Zip-loc snack bag)*

---

**LUNCH**
Mexican Potato:
½ cup Rosarita fat-free refried beans
1 tablespoon shredded cheddar cheese
4 oz. potato
Salsa

---

*Cook potato in microwave until soft. Top with beans and cheese. Cook in microwave for a short time to heat beans on potato. Fruit is a good side dish with this.*
**Snack**
Cheesy Corn Puffs:
1 cup puffed corn (in bag in market, cereal section, brand name "Pure & Simple" or "El Molino"--ingredients should say only "whole corn")
1 tablespoon fat-free grated Parmesan cheese
*Put puffed corn and Parmesan cheese in a paper bag and shake.*

---

**DINNER**
Clams Linguine:
2 oz. canned whole baby clams
2 tablespoons ricotta cheese made with skim milk
1 cup diced leek
1 teaspoon granulated garlic
Basil
1 cup linguine pasta

---

*Cook pasta. Heat ricotta in microwave. Fold clams, seasonings and cheese into the drained cooked pasta. Have a salad and 1 tablespoon fat-free dressing on the side.*
**Snack**
Baked Apple
1 apple
2 teaspoons 100% fruit jam (no sugar)
*Cook apple in microwave until soft. Put jam on top of apple to sweeten.*

*Your day was:*    Approximately 1,245 calories, 1,006 mg. sodium, and 152 mg. cholesterol
            20% protein                    66% carbohydrates                    14% fat

# Day 16

**Part I:**  No Stress "In"

**Part II:**  How Sweet It Is or Isn't

**Part III:**  Have the Sweet Look of
Success

## Just For You (<u>Y</u>our <u>O</u>wn <u>U</u>niqueness)

Have a date at a spa for a massage, manicure, pedicure, or facial.  You are worth it.  It is not a woman's thing, it is a pleasure for anyone.

# Day 16
## Part I:                       No Stress "In"

Stress is your reaction to an activity that affects your nervous system, blood pressure, heart rate and attitude, among other things. So how important is it to manage your stress levels? The dictionary defines stress: a strain or straining force exerted upon the body that tends to deform its shape, emphasis, importance and significance.

When you say "I am stressed out" or "really in stress," or you might say, "that person or situation really stresses me out"? Remember the definition states that this strain or force deforms the body. The definition never states that the stress changes the situation or solves the problem.

There is stress that stimulates you and is caused by a positive action. And, of course, the stress involved in growth experiences like school, weddings, competitions, to name a few. So there is negative stress as well as positive stress, but the body doesn't know the difference. It only reacts by constriction, pressure, acceleration and distortion. Enough stress on the body can cause such deformity as stroke, heart attack, or headache.

Your goal is to manage your life so that you let no stress "in." This means you let things unfold. A wise sage once said, "I will not be affected by victory or failure; these are but events on my path." Let my response to these events be simply *acceptance*. Just learn from each life event and move on. The following lists are (1) stress "in": symptoms of stress and (2) stress out: ways to reduce stress--ways to release stress:

## STRESS "IN"

Check the symptoms of stress exhaustion you've noticed lately in yourself. Here is a list of the stress "in" and what it causes in your life:

Exhaustion
___appetite change
___headaches
___tension
___fatigue
___insomnia
___weight change
___colds
___muscle aches
___digestive upsets
___pounding heart
___accident prone
___teeth grinding
___rash
___restlessness
___foot tapping
___finger drumming
___increased alcohol,
   drug, tobacco use

Emotional
___anxiety
___frustration
___the "blues"
___mood swings
___bad temper
___nightmares
___crying spells
___irritability
___"no one cares"
___depression
___nervous laugh
___worrying
___easily discouraged
___little joy

Spiritual
___emptiness
___loss of meaning
___doubt
___unforgiving
___martyrdom
___looking for magic
___loss of direction
___ needing to "prove"
   self
___cynicism
___apathy

Mental
___forgetfulness
___dull sense
___poor concentration
___low productivity
___negative attitude
___confusion
___lethargy
___whirling mind
___no new ideas
___boredom
___spacing out
___negative self-talk

Relational
___isolation
___intolerance
___resentment
___loneliness
___lashing out
___hiding
___clamming up
___lowered sex drive
___nagging
___distrust
___fewer contacts with friends
___lack of intimacy

**STRESS OUT**

**Reducing Stress**

1. Be prepared to wait.
2. Never arrange a meeting place that has no telephone.
3. Find the humor in a situation.
4. Keep a "busy kit" handy when you travel.
5. Relax your standards.
6. Get help with the jobs you dislike.
7. Establish a serene place of your own.
8. Change your perspective.
9. Count your blessings.
10. Carry a book in your car or purse.
11. Keep time fillers by the phone.
12. Memorize your favorite poems.
13. Keep a supply of individually wrapped sugar-free candy or sugar-free gum handy.
14. Travel light.
15. Be prepared for rain.
16. Ask questions.
17. Make contingency plans.
18. Unclutter your life.
19. Avoid reliance on chemical aids.
20. Listen to music.
21. Have a bulletin board by the phone for messages.

**Releasing Stress**

1. Get in touch with yourself.
2. Take time out.
3. Find enjoyable ways to exercise.
4. Get it off your chest.
5. Talk to a loving friend or relative.
6. Reward yourself after stressful activities.
7. Take leisurely baths
8. Schedule more activities that are fun.
9. Take a break from the children.
10. Have a massage.
11. Unwind before bedtime.
12. Read a book.
13. Do handcrafts you enjoy, dance, play, draw.
14. Play a game.

# Day 16
## Part II:            How Sweet It Is--Or Isn't

*"Just a spoonful of sugar helps the medicine go down."* The truth is that many food manufacturers think a spoonful or more of sugar helps a lot of foods go down. Therefore, it is common practice to add sugar to all types of foods. In fact, sugar usually accounts for one-fifth of Americans' total daily calories. That's an average of 12 tablespoons a day, which can add up to the average American consuming 128 pounds of sugar per year. That can be quite a sweet tooth!

Even people who do not have an attraction to sweets may be unaware of how much sugar they actually consume. Perhaps the sugar added to the morning coffee doesn't add up to much, but sugar is often "hidden" in many prepared items. It is present in large amounts in baked goods, breakfast cereals, ice cream, and even in processed meats (e.g., hot dogs and bologna, to name a few).

Reinforcements for eating sweets are everywhere. From childhood, we learned to "finish your dinner or you won't get dessert" or "if you are good, I'll give you a cookie." Television commercials and advertisements tempt us with delicious-looking sweets. Friends and relatives may say, "I made your favorite dessert" or "sweets for my sweet." It takes practice and preparation to decondition your taste buds and attitudes regarding sweets.

Although not directly responsible for certain health conditions, it is known that diets high in sugar can lead to tooth decay, obesity, heart disease, hypo- and hyperglycemia.

***Calorically Speaking:***          Sugar contains 4 calories per gram.
                                     1 teaspoon = 16 calories.

***Sugar is Sugar is Sugar:***
Sugar comes in many forms. Most notable is sucrose or white table sugar. It is also often used in other forms such as:

- honey
- molasses
- corn syrup
- brown sugar
- maple syrup
- raw sugar

There are less obvious sugars that are added to foods. They include:
- fructose
- glucose
- lactose
- maltose

To identify these sugars on product labels, look for the "ose" suffice. *Beware of labels claiming "sugar-free"*: Legally this only means it does not contain sucrose or table sugar. Watch for the disguised sugars.

***Check out the Sugar Hideaways***:

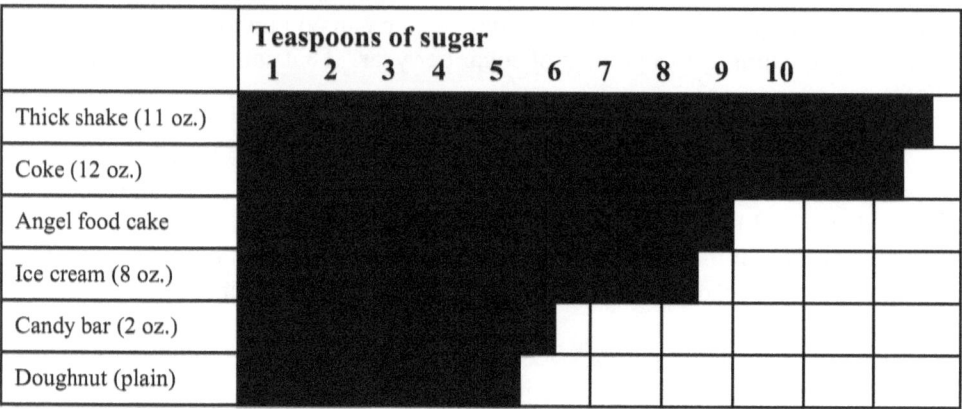

| | Teaspoons of sugar | | | | | | | | | |
| --- | --- | --- | --- | --- | --- | --- | --- | --- | --- | --- |
| | 1 | 2 | 3 | 4 | 5 | 6 | 7 | 8 | 9 | 10 |
| Thick shake (11 oz.) | | | | | | | | | | |
| Coke (12 oz.) | | | | | | | | | | |
| Angel food cake | | | | | | | | | | |
| Ice cream (8 oz.) | | | | | | | | | | |
| Candy bar (2 oz.) | | | | | | | | | | |
| Doughnut (plain) | | | | | | | | | | |

# Day 16
## Part III:     Have The Sweet Look Of Success

Who's the person with the clean, fresh look? You. As a successful person you are not just under obligation to live a good, conscientious life. Part of the bargain is that you look the part. Represent yourself with a good image in every way, including your wardrobe. Rich or poor, skinny or fat, tall or short, we are all faced with the same problem--how to choose the clothes that are most flattering. If you are rich and willowy, with the preferred combination of horizontals and verticals, your task is considerably easier. But many people who lack these resources possess a highly developed sense of fashion. Fashion know-how does not have to be inborn, it can be learned.

Your ability to choose your clothes can be sharpened by constant awareness and analysis of what is good fashion. Study fashion magazines, clothing ads, the window displays of better shops and smartly dressed people. Exposure to good fashion is an excellent teacher. Try to decide what makes an ensemble outstanding. Is it the becoming design of the style, the beautiful coordination of color, or the clever use of accessories? Look for new features--a change in sleeve, a hem line or collar, a jewelry fad, the set of the shoulders, a new shape? The person who is on the watch for fashion smartness finds many ideas that apply to his/her own wardrobe.

The essence of good taste in fashion is simplicity. Simplicity with a flair is quiet, uncluttered simplicity. Tasteful attire is never overdone, never offensively revealing in cut or fit, always appropriate to the occasion, person's personality, etc. Good taste is what is good for you; if it feels right, it probably is. Ask the "Boss."

The plus in fashion today is that you can choose any look, you are not restricted to what fashion dictates. This freedom is also a liability, for you must know how to create the total look. If you are wearing a period look such as the forties, you must coordinate the whole look from shoes to make-up, to hat and glove. The forecasts for fashion are wide open. Know your proportion, color and personal flair and you will always present your best self. If you've got it (what it takes to make a look), flaunt it.

The total look is individual art and it is here to stay. Accessories are in full bloom: gloves, hats, padded shoulders, custom jewelry, scarves, ties, lower heeled shoes and platforms, everything goes. The length of skirts and jackets are versatile. The days (in the 60's and 70's) of women not having a dress or a man not having a suit are over. There is a time in all of our lives when we will "dress" for the occasion. So be prepared, know when, where and how to dress.

Wishing will not make it so. However, if you do wish to appear chic, smart and attractive, go ahead, make that wish, but back it up with effort, knowledge and a confident attitude. Your results are based on the following:

- Be vain about your good points, vain enough to make the most of them.
- Keep your bad points a secret by choosing clothes that conceal them.
- Know your balance lines, those lines that flatter your body proportions.
- Use color to your advantage.
- Dress to suit the occasion or if you are not sure what the occasion is, wear something simple so it will not appear over or understated.

- Know it is never how much you spend, but how wisely and tastefully you spend that makes you well dressed.
- Use accessories to make a basic wardrobe outstanding and creative.

*Exercise:* (indoors 30 minutes)

Help From the Pros: Aerobic class on television.

*Insight/Action:*

Insight:

Action:

*Affirmation:*

If everything looks black...I've probably got my eyes closed.

# Menu Options
## "Fuel For the Day"

**BREAKFAST**

Hot Apple Oatmeal:

1 cup cooked plain oatmeal

½ cup skim or low-fat milk

½ teaspoon cinnamon

2 teaspoons 100% all fruit jam

½ cup diced apple

*Cut up apple and cook in microwave until soft and warm. Heat up oatmeal and put in jam to sweeten. Top oatmeal with cooked apples, cinnamon and milk.*

**Snack Boost**

2 dried apricots

3 unsalted almonds

*(in a Zip-loc snack bag)*

**LUNCH**

High-Burning Mac N Cheese:

1 cup cooked whole wheat macaroni

½ cup non-fat cottage cheese

3 tablespoons mozzarella cheese from skim milk

1 teaspoon mustard

*Cook macaroni. Top with cottage cheese, mix in mustard to taste, and mozzarella cheese. Add a fruit or vegetable or salad.*

**Snack**

Chocolate Soy Shake:

½ cup Westsoy Lite chocolate soy milk

½ banana

*Mix in blender until tall and frothy.*

**DINNER**

Sirloin Steak and Rice:

3 oz. sirloin steak (trimmed and grilled)

4 oz. yam (cooked in microwave until soft, season with cinnamon

1 cup steamed vegetables.

**Snack**

Frozen Grapes:

2 cups grapes

*Rinse grapes until clean. Place in freezer bag in the freezer overnight.*

***Your day was:*** Approximately 1,286 calories, 641 mg. sodium, and 94 mg. cholesterol

21% protein          64% carbohydrates          15% fat

# Day 17

**Part I:** **Create Positive Interactions with Others**

**Part II:** **Surviving "Time Out"**

**Part III:** **Life Is For Giving, Follow Your Bliss**

**Just For You (<u>Y</u>our <u>O</u>wn <u>U</u>niqueness)**

Create a personal collage of your dream wardrobe, use magazine pictures, fabric swatches and so on. Go all the way, get inspired.

# Day 17
## Part I:     Create Positive Interaction With Others

As you look at your life at this time, let go of negative traits and set in motion a new positive direction. You may meet people who are attuned to negative activity. They may tell you how wrong everything appears, they may even try to put you down for being a peaceful, happy person. While you may meet 20 positive people, a single crude, insensitive, loud-mouthed obnoxious person is enough to burst your bubble. How do you keep your attitude positive?

You succeed by not giving your attention to negative people. You do not have time. Anything they have to say, that is not upbeat, does not deserve your attention. Negative ideas do not deserve a place in your mind, because you experience what you give your attention to. It is a miracle to be alive; appreciate this miracle. Put your attention on good, on joy, on health.

Do not allow people who would discriminate against you to interfere with your progress today. They cannot affect you without your permission. Make a decision not to let yourself be involved with inappropriate encounters. Inappropriate encounters are those that support myths about you, your appearance, talents and attitudes. Remember, you are beautiful in every way and you need not feel threatened by anyone. If you argue with a fool, observers may not be able to tell the difference between you. When you have completely accepted yourself, there is no need for justification, comparison, or competition. You do not need to justify your value, either to yourself or to others. Flood your mind with positive declaration, images and feelings so that all the old shackles of negative thinking completely disappear. Let your attention be on only good and you will experience the same. Give attention to those in your life who give positive energy. Share quality time with them and your interaction will always be productive. Love each person, but give time to those who build rather than tear down.

### Help Others Bloom

Do not bury your own wonderfulness under harsh words. Act as if you are special, and, by God, you will be special! Similarly, respect the specialness in other people, too. If you have healed yourself, help others to heal themselves, too. If you have stopped hurting yourself, also stop hurting others. If you have restored yourself, restore others, too. If you have stopped depleting yourself, stop depleting others. Invite others to grow and flourish, and not shrivel and die.

People are always reacting to each other--positively, negatively, or passively. There are those who, by their very presence, make others feel important, alive, and capable of becoming someone better than they have ever known before. Be this kind of person.

As you help others bloom, you too will bloom. In giving to others, you are invariably giving to yourself as well. You cannot encourage someone to stand up against adversity without also committing yourself to be encouraged. You cannot encourage someone to be noble and charitable and remain ignoble and mean. As you give to others, you give to yourself, too. People need help to grow. We all yearn for continuous achievement and growth.

Be one of those magnificent people who invite others to grow, to encourage talents and unseen capacities to blossom forth and be known to the world. Robert Browning was such a person. His love was the breath of Elizabeth Barrett's life. He lifted her from a sickly, middle-aged invalid into an exquisite artist. You, too, can help others bloom.

# Day 17
# Part II:    Surviving "Time Out" (Special Events)

! Modify recipes to be lower in fat, sugar and salt.

! When you are responsible for food, always introduce low-fat alternatives.

! When someone else is handling food arrangements, offer your input or bring a low-fat dish.

! Avoid thoughtless eating:
  ⌒ Be mindful of finger foods.
  ⌒ Use newly developed stress management skills.
  ⌒ Practice time management techniques.
  ⌒ Plan your meals and preparation time.

! Don't leave munchies on the counter; put them away after serving. If this is not possible, stand away from buffet tables or snack bowls.

! Remember, you are always in charge of what you eat, regardless of other people's comments.

! Experiment with new ways to enjoy special occasions without overindulging.
  ∩ Get involved in conversation with someone you've just met.
  ∩ Be the life of the party.
  ∩ Try new games.

! At mealtime:
  ∩ Have a glass of water available, drink before the meal
  ∩ Use visualization, what do you want your plate to look like when it is full.
  ∩ Take small portions, since there are usually lots of choices.
  ∩ Eat slowly, enjoy the company around you.
  ∩ Be conscious of the number of calories added from alcoholic beverages.
  ∩ Before you take seconds, wait 20 minutes, then ask yourself, "Am I really hungry?"

! Deal with holiday foods at work by:
  ∩ Avoiding the areas where food is kept.
  ∩ Offering your coworkers delicious, low-fat treats.

! If you are overloaded with food gifts, consider giving them to extended family members, neighbors, friends and coworkers. Also consider requesting "healthy" gifts such as cookbooks, exercise outfits, vegetable steamers, exotic spices, pedometers, relaxation tapes, and "fruit of the month" clubs.

## Dining Out The Low-Fat Way

Americans love restaurant dining! In fact, 50% of American meals are eaten in restaurants. Because of this fact, Americans need assistance in learning to choose delicious foods that are also nutritious. *Remember, low-fat choices will usually contain fresh fruits and vegetables, grains and legumes.* Beware of how the food is prepared, since heavy batters or sauces can quickly increase calories and fat content. Learn which terms and phrases indicate low-fat and high-fat preparation styles.

**Keep an eye open for menu clues:**

| Low-Fat Terms | Low-Fat, but High in Sodium | High-Fat Terms |
|---|---|---|
| Steamed | Pickled | Buttery |
| In its own juice | In cocktail sauce | Sauteed |
| Garden fresh | Smoked | Fried |
| Broiled | In broth | Creamed |
| Roasted | In tomato base | Cheesy |
| Poached | | Alfredo |

**Here are some general tips for restaurant ordering:**

*Breakfast*
- Choose fresh fruit or juice.
- Choose whole grain bread toasted dry, with margarine or jam served on the side.
- Choose hot cereals such as oatmeal; be aware that many prepared cold cereals contain sugar and sodium.
- Limit eggs to 3 per week -- ask for poached or soft boiled or request only one yolk in an omelet.
- Choose waffles topped with fresh fruit and yogurt.

*Beverages*
- Choose fruit juices, sparkling water, tomato juice, iced tea, or water.
- Limit intake of alcoholic beverages.

*Appetizers*
- Choose "steamed" seafood, raw vegetables, fresh fruit, or corn tortillas.
- Ask that salted nuts, buttery crackers, and potato and tortilla chips be removed from the table.

*Entrees*
- Choose poultry, fish, shellfish and vegetable dishes.
- Choose lean red meat periodically.
- Choose items that are broiled, baked, poached, roasted, or steamed.

*Salads*
- Ask your server what items are included in the salad (cheese, eggs, meat, bacon, and croutons can really boost the fat content).
- Order all dressings on the side, so you can control the amount used. Try fresh lemon juice as an all-purpose flavor enhancer.

*Desserts/Coffee*
- Choose fresh fruits, fruit ices, sherbets or angel food cake.
- Be wary of dairy substitutes, such as non-dairy creamers. These are frequently made with high saturated fat bases such as coconut or palm oil.

# Day 17
# Part III:    Life Is For Giving, Follow Your Bliss

Learning how to live creatively ultimately means learning how to work creatively. Your work should not be a mere grind to earn money. Your work should touch the core of your personality. Only when you work at the things you enjoy does work offer you a channel for self-improvement, growth, exultation.

Your first task, then, is to find out what you enjoy doing that is of service and that can earn money. If you think work is a grind, then you are doing the wrong kind of work and must plan on doing something that has personal meaning for you. Failure to work in something you enjoy will drain all your initiative, courage and hope. Work is an opportunity for you to fulfill your self-expression.

Only those people who love their work achieve true success. Did you know that only five percent of Americans love their work? Most people lead mediocre lives because they do not enjoy what they do. When your heart is not in your tasks, then no amount of effort is going to last long enough to bring you the success you desire. Choose your work well, for that is where you spend 75 percent of your waking, quality hours.

Thomas Edison loved his work, and that is why he was able to succeed so brilliantly as an inventor. As a mark of his enthusiasm, he left, at the time of his death, some 2500 notebooks crammed with notes of his work and ideas.

It is a fine thing to work hard, for effort creates, but without love for your work, you will not be able to summon up sufficient enthusiasm to work well. Within each of us is that special thing, that talent that we are to give. The philosopher Joseph Campbell refers to this activity as your bliss. To find it, sit quietly, alone, and ask yourself what it is I am to do. Your inner voice will answer, this is why work is called a vocation, a call; follow it, for it is only for you to do. Life is for giving; follow your bliss.

Exercise:

    Help from Pros:  Complimentary visit to local gym.

*Insight/Action:*

Insight:

Action:

*Affirmation:Free Yourself!*

    *Work like you don't need moneoy, love like you've never been hurt and dance like no ones' watching.*

# Menu Options
## "Fuel For the Day"

| **BREAKFAST** | |
|---|---|
| Egg Burrito: | |
| ½ cup Eggbeaters | Diced tomatoes |
| 1 tablespoon cheese | Vegetable spray |
| Salsa to taste | Whole wheat tortilla |

*Scramble up Eggbeaters in non-stick pan sprayed with vegetable spray (e.g., Pam). Put in tortilla on top of Eggbeaters while cooking. Put top on fry pan for a few seconds ((to heat tortilla). Put tortilla on a plate filled with Eggbeaters, cheese and tomatoes. Add salsa to taste. Eat a fruit to balance this meal (grapefruit, orange, cantaloupe, etc.).*

**Snack Boost**
Fruit

| **LUNCH** |
|---|
| Tuna Pita: |
| 1 whole wheat pita bread |
| 3 oz. tuna packed in water (drained) |
| 1 tablespoon fat-free mayonnaise |
| Lettuce and tomato |

*Mix tuna with mayonnaise. Fill pita with tuna mixture and lettuce and tomato. Have a fruit on the side.*

**Snack**
Celery with Peanut Butter:
2 stalks of celery, each stalk filled with 2 teaspoons Laura Scudder's unsalted natural peanut butter

| **DINNER** |
|---|
| Sloppy Susan: |
| ¼ cup ground turkey |
| ¼ cup tomato sauce |
| 1 teaspoon chili powder |
| 1/8 cup diced onions |
| 1 whole wheat hamburger bun |

*Brown onions and ground turkey in non-stick pan. Add tomato sauce and simmer for 5 minutes. Serve over open-faced hamburger bun with a salad.*

**Snack**
Fruit

***Your day was:*** Approx. 1,203 calories, 2,151 mg. sodium, and 88 mg. cholesterol
25% protein                55% carbohydrates                20% fat

137

# Day 18

**Part I:**    **You Are A Wonder In the World**

**Part II:**   **Program Yourself for Success**

**Part III:**  **Build a Support Network**

### Just For You (<u>Y</u>our <u>O</u>wn <u>U</u>niqueness)

Do something that seems silly, that takes you back to your
childhood or youth.  Example:  play jacks with a child.

# Day 18
## Part I:       You Are A Wonder In The World

Yesterday, you learned to express a child-like attitude of self-acceptance. Now, for the rest of your life, reinforce that child, build it up. Continually touch the heart of your own power. When you do this, you create a magnetic circle of self-confidence around you. People are attracted to your sense of specialness, they will want to be around you, unconsciously hoping that some of your magic will rub off on them too.

You must see yourself as accomplished, as capable of easily learning new tasks. Remember you are the gifted one, the special one. You are a wonder in the world. All of creation can never come up with another you. Accept your specialness, embrace it, live in it. You are the king or queen of your universe, yourself.

You may feel rather ordinary; and as long as you feel this way, you will be ordinary, and people will treat you as ordinary.

You should "act as if" you are extraordinary, as if your life really matters, as if you have a divine mission here on earth. If you do this, you will become extraordinary. People will expect great things from you. You will expect great things from yourself.

You will find life exciting, magical. Once you rid yourself of excuses, once you throw off that dowdy self-image, which kept you safely locked into mediocrity, you will have to do things, you will have to perform, and you will have to be a smashing success. Do not be afraid of this...for this will be the real you, the you who had been buried under criticism. Remove the poison of self-criticism from your system. Be special NOW.

# Day 18
## Part II:  Program Yourself for Success

**What You Say To Yourself**

| Problem Category | Negative Monologues | Appropriate Monologues |
|---|---|---|
| **1. Losing pounds** | "I'm not losing fast enough." "I've starved myself and haven't lost a thing." "I've been more consistent than Mary and she is losing faster than I am.  It isn't fair." | |
| **2. Capabili-ties** | "I just don't have the will power." "I'm just naturally fat." "Why should this work?  Nothing else has." "I'll probably just regain it." "What the heck--I'd rather be fat than miserable; besides, I'm not that heavy." | |

| | | |
|---|---|---|
| **3. Excuses** | "If it weren't for my job, my family...I could lose weight."<br>"It's just impossible to eat right with a schedule like mine."<br>"I'm just so nervous all the time--I have to eat to satisfy my needs."<br>"Maybe tomorrow, next week, next year." | |
| **4. Goals** | "Well, there goes my diet.  That coffee cake probably cost me two pounds, and after I told myself no more sweets!"<br>"I always blow it on the weekends."<br>"Fine, I went off my diet, I may as well enjoy myself today." | |
| **5. Food Thoughts** | "I can't stop thinking about food."<br>"When I see or think about food I have to have it." | |

## I am a Kaleidoscope

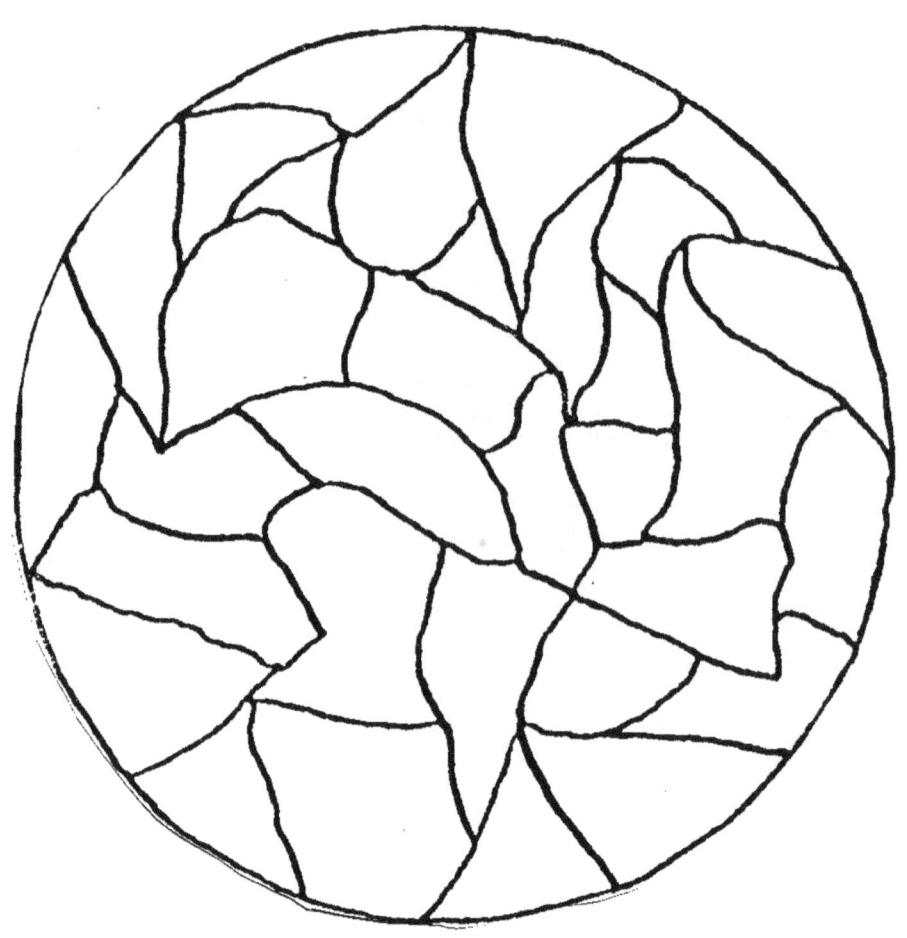

Write all of your qualities, talents, skills, resources  in the chips of the
kaleidoscope.  Remember, all of these traits are inside you.  Program
yourself from the inside out. Make pictures by moving on purpose.
It's in you...

Old ideas I have released:

New ideas of self:

# Day 18
## Part III:        Build a Support Network

Support people are special. Many people tend to minimize how difficult it is to lose weight and make lifestyle changes. Your support people have not only acknowledged this difficulty, but they have taken on the demands of being a friend through thick and thin. Here are some helpful hints on how to maintain successful, rewarding support relationships.

1.    *A Little Encouragement Goes a Long Way*
    Tell your support people that you appreciate them.

2.    *Kind Reminders Can Only Help*
    If you feel that a support person is losing focus of your goals and needs, make suggestions as to how you feel he can best help you.

3.    *Ask for Help*
    Only when you communicate can someone offer you assistance. If no one knows there's a problem they can't help.

4.    *Rewards Are . . . Rewarding*
    Just as you enjoy and value rewards, so do your support people. Give your support people a pat, a hug, a gift, a thank-you.

5.    *A Walk In Your Lifestyle Can Be Enlightening*
    Ask a support person to buddy with you for a day of low-fat eating or exercise. Sharing behaviors can increase interpersonal commitment and understanding.

**Redefining Social Support Needs**

Social support needs change as your lifestyle changes. Now that you have created realistic goals for yourself and understand what it involves to change behaviors, it is a good time to reassess your social support needs. Through the course of the program you have probably discovered that you need more support in some areas, less in others and some in ways that you never thought of. Use the questions below to help you clarify your current social support needs. Discuss your responses with your support network.

1. What behavior changes am I having difficulty with? How can someone help me progress?

2. Do I need more encouragement to exercise or make appropriate food choices? If "yes," what type of support do I need?

3. How has my self-image changed? Do I feel more empowered now? How do my answers to these questions affect my social support needs?

4. Is my support network directing me or supporting me? How do I respond when I get advice? Am I happy with my response?

*Exercise:*

Help from the Pros: Day at the "Y" (YMCA) facility -- call ahead.

*Insight/Action:*

Insight:

Action:

*Affirmation:*

I let go of yesterday and embrace today with love.

# Menu Options
## "Fuel For the Day"

**BREAKFAST**
1 cup Special K cereal (not strawberry)
2 teaspoons 100% all fruit jam
1 tablespoon sliced unsalted almonds
½ banana

½ cup skim or low-fat milk   *Put all ingredients in a bowl.*

**Snack Boost**
2 dried apricots
3 unsalted almonds
*(in a Zip-loc snack bag)*

**LUNCH**
Healthy Guacamole:

2-ounce slice of avocado                    1/8 cup diced tomatoes
½ cup non-fat cottage cheese Salsa to taste
1 slice whole wheat tortilla

*Mash the avocado with the cottage cheese and stir in diced tomatoes and salsa. Place on top of warmed whole wheat tortilla. Eat with a vegetable or fruit.*

**Snack**
Fruit

**DINNER**
Chicken Cacciatore:
3 oz. baked skinless chicken breast
1 cup cooked linguine
¼ cup meatless spaghetti sauce
*Cover baked chicken and linguine pasta with spaghetti sauce. Have a green salad with 1 tablespoon low-fat salad dressing on the side.*

**Snack**
Baked Apple
1 apple
2 teaspoons 100% fruit jam (no sugar)
*Cook apple in microwave until soft. Put jam on top of apple to sweeten.*

*Your day was:*   Approximately 1,181 calories, 1,376 mg. sodium, 169 mg. cholesterol
24% protein                    54% carbohydrates                    22% fat

# Day 19

**Part I:**      **Take Time For Yourself**

**Part II:**     **Create a Fashion Network**

**Part III:**    **Have A Vision, A Life Purpose**

## Just For You (<u>Y</u>our <u>O</u>wn <u>U</u>niqueness)

Read a chapter in a book that you have wanted to read but didn't feel that you have the time. Just open it and read a chapter.

# Day 19
## Part I:                    Take Time For Yourself

Take time for yourself each day, time to communicate with your best
friend, you. You need at least one hour in twenty four to care for yourself. Give
yourself a nap, read a book, go for a walk, but enjoy the time. We sometimes say
we just do not have time to eat right or groom ourselves or shop. Look at the
truth about time. We have 168 hours a week. We prioritize our use of it with
what we think is important to our survival. Is it approval from others,
acceptance, promise for a job well done, fear about loosing face that drives you
to loose time? Examine your motives for your activities and put you into your
life. Are you worth one hour out of 24? Give yourself that one hour a day. You
will love yourself for that gift. Remember, you can eat an elephant, one bite at a
time. The time you give yourself will change your life.

### *Prioritize Your Time*

You are aware of your strengths, potentials, your image of yourself,
others' image of you, your body design and so on. When you devote a great
portion of your life to a single purpose, such as expressing an ideal image, you
tend to lose pieces of the other parts of your life that make you whole. You must
balance your life by including all aspects of your life. Much of your life depends
upon how you coordinate your life activities. You will find that you can get
everything done if you prioritize and organize your time. In order to be
successful in coordinating your life, consider the following:

- Coordinate time
- Organize a schedule of activities
- Clear away clutter, old "stuff" that you are not using
- Discipline yourself
- Work smarter, not harder

Do not forget there are 168 hours in the week for everyone. Some make
it a successful money making love adventure, while others cry because they do
not have enough time. Prioritize your life and time. Above all, take time for
yourself. Coordinate your eating schedule, you will see the weight go It's your
new weigh. .

# Day 19
## Part II:                     Create a Fashion Network

The accessories that you select, and the way that you wear them, reveal your personality, in particular, your creativity and sense of fashion. Some people can turn a simple outfit into something fashionable by the way they use accessories. The difference between one's shirt or dress, and another's, may just be a marvelous belt or a stylish tie. Smart accessories are a wise investment. Here is where you can have fun, wear fads and be creative. Wear accessories with flair and with daring. Do not just put it on, make a statement.

### Camouflage

You can use positive camouflage through dressing. The outfit you wear can compliment or detract. Do not play up your faults, but capitalize on your assets. Light makes larger, dark makes smaller. For example, with small hips and large shoulders, wear a dark top.

Also, broken lines make short and unbroken lines make long. So, short people look fine in one color from top to hem, while tall folks wear two colors well.

Further, bulky, textured fabrics make heavy, smooth, lightweight textures appear light. (However, texture and bulk can look rich).

Use these camouflage theories to your advantage, but be creative and do not get stuck in a stereotypical dressing habit. Use a full length mirror to test the look. Listen for reactions from others and evaluate positively. Use your wardrobe to create a fashion network.

# Day 19
## Part III:          Have A Vision, A Life Purpose

If you were a hundred (100) years old and being interviewed by a newspaper reporter who wanted to know about your life, how would you want to describe what you have achieved? Now is the time to look at your life, define your vision, your purpose. Deep within you is the knowledge, the realization that your life has a purpose, a destiny, a meaning which must be discovered and pursued. Until this is accomplished, you may experience boredom, dissatisfaction, frustration, the feeling of vague emptiness.

Answer these questions:

1. What do you think are some typical purposes for living?
2. What do worthwhile purposes have as components?
3. What can you do to make the world a better place?
4. Do you have a vision, a purpose in life?

**Exercise:**

Think about your vision/purpose. Brainstorm using the answers above. Take into consideration your dreams, talents, interests and the values that you practice. There are no limitations. If you can conceive of the idea, it is yours. Believe that there are no obstacles but those that you create and anything that a creator creates can be un-created by its creator. You may feel that you need more time to think about your purpose.

This is not true, for you can change and modify it at any time. But by deciding on something right now, you will be 1) making a decision; 2) writing it down; 3) taking the first steps, taking action. So write down your purpose, be specific. After writing your purpose, go to the next steps.

How will your purpose affect:

1. Your life?
2. The lives of others?
3. Global concerns?

I have a new attitude; I believe in myself. I'm over weight.

*Exercise:*

Help from the Pros: Video exercise program.

*Insight/Action:*

Insight:

Action:

*Affirmation: You may be disappointed if you fail, but you are doomed if you don't try. Beverly Sills*

# Menu Options
## "Fuel For the Day"

| BREAKFAST |
| --- |
| Creamy P.B. & J.: |
| 1 tablespoon Laura Scudder's Natural peanut butter |
| 1 tablespoon ricotta cheese made with skim milk |
| 2 teaspoons Smucker's Simply Fruit jam (100% fruit, no sugar) |
| 1 slice of whole wheat bread |

*Spread peanut butter, cheese and jam on whole wheat bread. Enjoy one cup cubed cantaloupe on the side.*
### Snack Boost
Fruit

| LUNCH |
| --- |
| Turkey Sandwich: |
| 2 slices of fresh unsalted turkey |
| ½ teaspoon of mustard |
| Lettuce and tomato |
| Between 2 slices of whole wheat bread |
| Fruit |

### Snack
Cheesy Corn Puffs:
1 cup puffed corn (in bag in market, cereal section, brand name "Pure & Simple" or "El Molino"--ingredients should say only "whole corn")
1 tablespoon fat-free grated Parmesan cheese
*Put puffed corn and Parmesan cheese in a paper bag and shake.*

| DINNER |
| --- |
| Spaghetti and Meat Sauce: |
| ¾ cup whole wheat pasta |
| ¼ cup cooked ground turkey |
| ¼ cup spaghetti sauce (Classico or Bertolli) without meat |

*Cook pasta in a sauce pan. Drain and top with heated spaghetti sauce and cooked ground turkey. Green salad with 1 tablespoon low-fat salad dressing.*
### Snack
Chocolate Shake:
3 oz. Westsoy Lite chocolate soy milk
½ banana
*Mix in a blender until tall and frothy.*

*Your day was:* Approximately 1,271 calories, 2,201 mg. sodium, 133 mg. cholesterol

| 21% protein | 60% carbohydrates | 19% fat |
| --- | --- | --- |

# Day 20

**Part I:**      **Build Self-Confidence**

**Part II:**     **The Last Word:  Acknowledge Your Specialness**

**Part III:**    **Be In Tune With Nature**

## Just For You (<u>Y</u>our <u>O</u>wn <u>U</u>niqueness)

Do something you don't like to do, just for discipline. Examples: Organize drawers, put old pictures in photo album.

# Day 20
## Part I:                    Build Self-Confidence

What is self-confidence?  Self-confidence is knowing who you are and loving that person.  Our culture teaches us to put ourselves last.  When you do, you are experiencing everyone's life but your own.  You are busy seeking acceptance, approval and recognition outside yourself.  You seek these things from others because you have never come to you.  You are starving to be a whole person, not realizing that you are already whole, you were born that way.  However, because you may feel that everyone is more valuable than you, you become other centered, outer directed.  The great goal in your life is to be you, to express your talents, skills, abilities and beauty.  It is your gift to the planet.  Self-confidence is built on the premise that you know and love yourself, moving with assurance and authority.

Today, you will look at ways to build self-confidence.  We are not advocating an egotistical attitude, on the contrary.  When you know yourself you can give to others in honest and beautiful ways.  You will want to be aware of who you are at all times.  I am honest.  Confidence about yourself allows you to give to others unconditionally.  You can develop a higher degree of confidence and self-esteem by having a clear image (sight) of yourself.  This is done first by identifying your strengths and potentials.  Second, by clearing out all of the myths (attitudes that limit your progress), and old beliefs about yourself.  Third, by practicing positive visualization.  Seeing what you want by picturing your goals, activities and ideal personality traits.  Finally, through action, being the person that you desire to be.  Keep your spirit high by putting your attention on your best self.  Practice the presence.  Remember, when defined, presence is pre--to bring forth, essence your unique life energy, your personal power.  So practice the presence at all times and you will experience self-confidence. Complete the following:

### Build Self-Confidence

Answer these questions for yourself:

1.    How does your concern over what another person might think of you affect your self-confidence?

2.    How does the fear of failure affect people's lives?  How about yours?

3.       In what ways do you compare yourself with others?  How does it affect your self-confidence?

4.       In what ways do you run yourself down?  How does this affect your self-confidence?

5.       In what situations do you have self-confidence?  What are some of the ways you lack self-confidence?  How are the two different?

6.       Do you have feelings of inferiority that affect your self-confidence?

7.       Conventional wisdom has it that a good deal of thinking about ourselves and our abilities is negative.

8.       By discussing these feelings, do you think you can do something to overcome them?  What?

9.       By acting self-confident you feel self-confident.

10.     How can you use affirmations to build self-confidence?

# Day 20
## Part II:              The Last Word:
## Acknowledge Your Specialness

*"I Am Special."*

*I'm special!!! In all the world there is no one like me.  Since the beginning of time, there has never been another person like me.  Nobody has my smile, nobody has my eyes, my nose, my hair, my hands, and my voice.  I'm special.  No one can be found who has my handwriting.  Nobody anywhere has my tastes--for food, music or art.*

*In all of time there has been no one who laughs like me, no one who cries like me.  And what makes me laugh and cry will never provoke identical laughter and tears from anybody else, ever. No one reacts to any situation just as I would react. I'm special.*

*I am the only one in all of creation who has my set of abilities. Oh, there will always be somebody who is better at one of the things I am good at, but no one in the universe can reach the quality of my combination of talents, ideas, abilities and feelings. Like a room of musical instruments, some may excel alone, but none can match the symphony sound when all are played together. I am special. I am rare.*

*And in rarity there is great value. Because of my great rare value, I need not attempt to imitate others. I will accept--yes, celebrate--my differences.*

*I am special. And I am beginning to see that I was made special for a purpose. There is a job for me that no one else can do as well as me. Out of all the billions of applicants, only one is qualified, only one has the right combination of what it takes.*

*That one is me. Because...I am special.*

--Author unknown

1.    In what ways are you special?

2.    Who are you?

3.    How do you express your own uniqueness?

4.    In what ways do you orchestrate your special qualities?

- Fashion Image
- Health
- Communication
- Personality

5.    Ask four people to answer these questions for you. You can then see how you are expressing your specialness.

# Day 20
## Part III:                Be In Tune With Nature

We live in a universe of order and beauty.  Each of our lives is a finite expression of the universe.  We live out of balance when we are not in tune with nature or the natural environment around us.  It is true that we create our environment by our essence or unique personal life.  What contributes to that uniqueness is our attitude, emotions, state of mind and love for others.  This has been stated over and over in this 21 day experience.  However, just as important to the contributions of our personal environment is the following:

     color - creates emotion, state of mind

     aroma - creates sensation, neuro communication

     music - creates mood, healing, emotion

     vitamins - create a balance in the mineral health of your body

Be attentive to taking in only pure food, water and air.  Food additives, even when judged harmless, on the large scale can create metabolic imbalances.  Avoid strenuous physical exertion and stay out of the direct sun for long periods of time.

Enjoy nature's beauty as often as possible.  Enjoy the sunrise, sunset, moonlit walks and natural settings like the ocean, forest and parks.  Be quiet, listen to nature speak to you through the birds, wind, rustling leafs on the trees and rushing brooks.  Look at the stars, animals and natural wonders.  Appreciate nature.  Try this exercise, go for a walk, and appreciate nature.  This activity grounds you and balances your body.  Do not look at nature as separate from you, be in tune with it.

***Exercise:***
Help from the Pros:  Visit a recreation exercise class in your city (plan ahead).

***Insight/Action:***

<u>Insight</u>:

<u>Action</u>:

***Affirmation:***

I accept myself unconditionally.

# Menu Options
## "Fuel For the Day"

---

**BREAKFAST**

Healthy Egg Muffin:
½ cup Eggbeaters
1 tablespoon shredded cheddar cheese
1 sliced beefsteak tomato
1 whole wheat English muffin (split)
Pepper to taste

---

*Cook up Eggbeaters in nonstick pan (sprayed with vegetable spray). Sprinkle cheddar cheese on top of Eggbeaters. Toast English muffin. Top muffin with tomato, Eggbeaters and cheese, and enjoy. Have a fruit on the side.*

**Snack Boost**

Fruit

---

**LUNCH**

Bean and Cheese Burrito:
½ cup Rosarita fat-free refried beans
1 tablespoon low-fat shredded cheddar cheese
1 whole wheat tortilla
*Spoon beans into tortilla. Sprinkle cheese on top of beans. Roll up tortilla. Heat in microwave for 2 minutes on high. Have a green salad with five small cooked shrimp and 1 tablespoon fat-free salad dressing*

---

**Snack**

Celery with Peanut Butter:
2 stalks of celery, each stalk filled with 2 teaspoons Laura Scudder's unsalted natural peanut butter

---

**DINNER**

Turkey Burger
3 oz. ground turkey patty
Mrs. Dash seasoning
Lettuce and tomato
1 whole wheat hamburger bun
*Fry turkey patty in a nonstick pan sprayed with vegetable spray. Place between a bun with lettuce, tomato and mustard. Eat with cole slaw.*
*Cole Slaw: ½ cup shredded cabbage mixed with 1 tablespoon fat-free mayonnaise and mustard (to taste)*

---

**Snack**

Frozen Grapes:
2 cups grapes
*Rinse grapes until clean. Place in a freezer bag in the freezer overnight.*

***Your day was:*** Approximately 1,288 calories, 2,264 mg. sodium, 98 mg. cholesterol
21% protein          56% carbohydrates          23% fat

# Day 21

**Part I:**    **Today Is The Best Day Of Your Life**

**Part II:**    **Write Your Success Story**

**Part III:**    **You Are Over Weight**

## Just For You (Your Own Uniqueness

Buy yourself a small plant.  Let it represent the new you.
Watch it grow as you grow.

# Day 21
## Part I:      Today Is The Best Day Of Your Life

It is time to say, "Farewell!" You have been given many ideas and invested many hours of time thinking about them, even applying them. You now have the rest of your life to reap the benefit of what you have learned. If you have opened your mind and your heart to the concepts expressed to you, you will now see yourself and your life ahead, in a larger dimension. You will realize that your limitations and barriers to personal effectiveness are self-imposed. You will have created an appetite for continued development of your mind, body and spirit. From here on, it is up to you.

You know, by now, that your life is created in the mind, out of your thoughts. You will experience what you create in your thoughts. Making life a fulfilling, exhilarating experience is dependent on the amount of diligence and effort you put forth to build a positive set of thoughts, beliefs and feelings.

Your life will be shaped by what you are and what you do. You will learn what you live. The principles that you have expressed and thought about do bring results if they are practiced. You may even want to set yourself the task of going for another 21 days, and keeping notes on how you applied the principle each day. Your life will be an incredibly more glorious adventure if it extends from positive attitudes, rather than thoughts of indifference and pessimism. Continue your journey of self-improvement and development. Today is the best day of your life and tomorrow will be even better, if you choose.

# Day 21
## Part II:      Write Your Success Story

You have participated in a 21-day experience, activities, exercises, and resources that you have used to get "over weight." Whether this was time wasted or time well spent is up to you. If you take these final words as a beginning rather than an ending, it will have been time invested wisely. You now have the rest of your life to reap the returns of the time invested in this experience.

If you have opened your mind and your heart to the concepts set forth, you will now see yourself and your life ahead in a larger dimension. You will realize that your limitations and barriers are self-imposed. You will experience success day by day, one day at a time. Please write your success story. Write your accomplishments, your goals, your vision, and how you succeeded.

**Success Story**

# Day 21
## Part III:                    You Are Over Weight

Congratulations!  Of all the things to get over, weight is the most
rewarding.  No other challenges are connected to life so directly.  If you are an
alcoholic, you can avoid alcohol, you do not need it to live.  The same is true of
drugs, smoking and other habits.  You can give them up and live but you cannot
give up eating and live.  The most important factor in overcoming weight is
knowing yourself, who you are.  You are a radiant, unique individual, one of a
kind.  Rather than focusing on your weight, you are putting your attention on
your assets, your strengths, your potentials.  These qualities represent your
essence, your special inner traits, and your attitude.  They represent who you are.
Your attitude comes from what you believe about yourself.  Remember to
practice living one moment at a time as discussed previously.  You can overcome
anything that you choose.  You can get over weight.  Fly free, discover Y.O.U.,
your own uniqueness, you are "over weight."

*Exercise:*

Help from the Pros:  Go out dancing.

*Insight/Action:*

Insight:

Action:

*Affirmation:*

I enjoy the present.  It is life's magnificent gift to me.

# Menu Options
## "Fuel For the Day"

**BREAKFAST**

Egg Burrito:

| | |
|---|---|
| ½ cup Eggbeaters | Diced tomatoes |
| 1 tablespoon cheese | Vegetable spray |
| Salsa to taste | Whole wheat tortilla |

*Scramble up Eggbeaters in non-stick pan sprayed with vegetable spray (e.g., Pam). Put in tortilla on top of Eggbeaters while cooking. Put top on fry pan for a few seconds ((to heat tortilla). Put tortilla on a plate filled with Eggbeaters, cheese and tomatoes. Add salsa to taste. Eat a fruit to balance this meal (grapefruit, orange, cantaloupe, etc.)*

**.Snack Boost**

1 Fruit

**LUNCH**

Chicken Pasta Salad:

| | |
|---|---|
| 1 cup cooked whole wheat macaroni | ½ cup cooked diced chicken |
| 1 tablespoon fat-free mayonnaise | ½ cup grapes |
| 2 tablespoons diced celery | 2 tablespoons diced green onions |
| 2 tablespoons diced tomatoes | Mrs. Dash seasoning |

*Mix al of the above ingredients in a bowl and enjoy.*

**Snack**

½ cup Knudsen's fat-free cottage cheese
¼ cup canned pineapple in water packed in a can

**DINNER**

3 oz. broiled salmon (with lemon and Mrs. Dash)
Yam (cooked in microwave until soft)

Salad with 1 tablespoon non-fat dressing

**Snack**

Blueberry Cream Cheese Parfait:

| | |
|---|---|
| 1 cup blueberries (fresh or frozen) | 2 tablespoons Cool Whip Lite |
| 1 tablespoon Philadelphia Light cream cheese | 1 teaspoon vanilla |

*Fold together all ingredients and serve in a bowl. Makes 1 serving.*

***Your day was:*** Approximately 1,230 calories, 1,269 mg. sodium, and 118 mg. cholesterol

| | | |
|---|---|---|
| 28% protein | 53% carbohydrates | 19% fat |

# Resources

# 21 Days of Menu Options

## Breakfasts
Cheesy Fruit Danish
Creamy Peanut Butter and Jelly
Hot Apple Oatmeal
Egg Burrito
Healthy Egg Muffin
Peanut Butter and Banana Rice
Cakes
Vegetable Omelet

## Lunches or Dinners
Tuna Sandwich
Mexican Stuffed Potato
Turkey Sandwich
Bean and Cheese Burrito
Healthy Guacamole
Sloppy Susan
Curried Chicken Stuffed Potato
Spaghetti with Meat Sauce
Halibut with Rice
Tuna Pita
Chicken Cacciatore
High-burning Mac and Cheese
Soup and Sandwich
Broiled Salmon and Yam
Sirloin Steak and Yam
Chicken Pita
Cheese Shrimp Pizza
Broccoli Tuna Melt
Chicken Pasta Salad
Turkey Burger
Shrimp Kabob
Egg Salad Sandwich
Baked Chicken and Yam
Mexican Potato
Clams Linguine
Sirloin Steak and Rice
Steak Bowl
Turkey Waldorf Salad Sandwich

## Snacks
Strawberry, Chocolate or Vanilla
Shake
Cheesy Corn Puffs
Snack Boost (almonds and dried
apricots)
Veggies & Dip
Cream Cheese Muffin and Jam
Cottage Cheese & Fruit
Fruit
Blueberry Cheesecake Parfait
Celery with Peanut Butter
Baked Apple
Jam Muffin and Hot Cocoa
Corn Puffs & Almonds
Frozen Grapes

# Shopping List

## Dairy Products

Skim or Low Fat Milk
Knudsen's Fat Free Cottage Cheese
Non fat Plain Yogurt
Egg Substitute or Egg Whites
Knudsen's Fat Free Sour Cream

## Meats &Fish

Chicken
Ground Turkey
Tuna, Halibut
Sirloin Steak
Clams, Shrimp

## Breakfast Foods

Plain Oatmeal
Special K Cereal
Wheat Germ
Puffed Corn

## Cheese/Dairy

Ricotta Fat Free Cheese
Cheddar, String, Parmesan, Mozzarella
Light Cream Cheese   Cool Whip Lite

## Canned  Vegetables/Fruits

Stewed Tomatoes
50% less salt Kidney Beans
Tomato Sauce
 Mexican Stewed Tomatoes
Pineapple Chunks

## Pasta & Rice

Brown Rice, wild rice
Whole Wheat Noodles
Whole Wheat  Pasta
Linguine

## Snacks

Peanut Butter
Smucker's Simply Fruit Jam (100%)
Almonds, dried apricots
Unsalted sunflower seeds,  walnuts

## Beverages

Water, Water, Water
Crystal Light
Swiss Miss Diet Coco, coffee /tea

A sample shopping only.  Make list from menu ideas.

# Acknowledgements

You have completed this 21-day experience. It draws from many resources in order to build a way of thinking, an attitude and a lifestyle that support overcoming the obsessive behavior related to weight. It draws from Psychology, Metaphysics, Ayurvedic science and the Total Image Program Series (TIPS). Thank you for the nutrition data and menu ideas contributed by Susan Hoag Stophel, Clinical Nutritionist.

I appreciate the sciences that have been used as references in this project. It is true, there is always a new weigh!

# About the Nutritionist

Susan Hoag Stophel has developed eating and nutritional programs for Carnation Health and Nutrition Centers and the Medical Wellness Center. She has taught at Learning Tree University and California Lutheran University. Ms. Stophel has written *The Ten Lb. Loss Challenge and Beyond* program (100,000 copies published by Women's Workout World based in Chicago, with 22 locations across the United States). She has written *Four Ingredients to Turn Up The Burn*, published by Denlinger's Publishing.

# An Invitation

You may have read this book out of curiosity. Consider yourself embarking on a new adventure, a path that can literally transform your life! The information now at your fingertips can re-educate your concept of transforming your image.

This book is designed through years of research, and is complemented by a remarkable hands-on seminar called Transform Your Image, Transform Your Life. This is an exciting six-hour experience, filled with experiences that can create a new you and support your resolve to transform your image.

After applying these techniques for 21 days, you will find you are free of the struggle and disappointments associated with weight. Embrace your horizons, stand tall; you are now in charge of your life. You are the "Boss." For more information about the seminar, you are invited to e-mail Dr. Sheard at cass4tlc@yahoo.com.

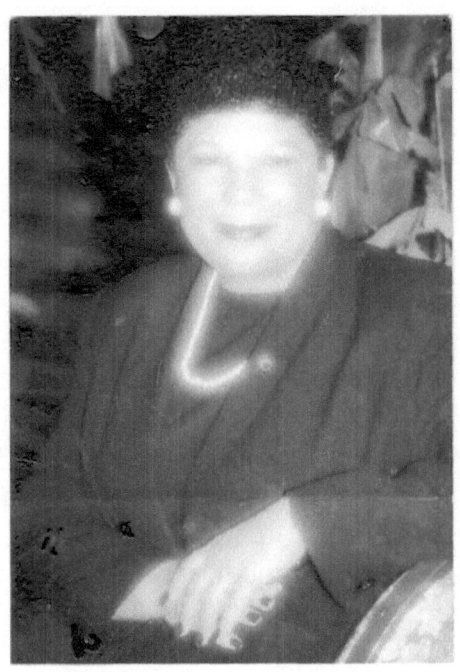

# About the Author

Dr. Ruinese Sheard, president of Transformation Life Connections (TLC) and creator of the TIPS system, is a Behavior/Life Strategist with thirty years' experience as a professional in personal and group transformation. These professions include counselor, educator, and project administrator. She has had experience as behavior/strategist and educator with Kaiser Permanente, as an image consultant, and charm instructor at Sears's stores and her own Cassandra's Image Center. Sheard was named Nordstrom's Woman Achiever of the Year and is listed in *Who's Who in Women in the United States*. She has authorized two personal growth books with featured workbooks and seminars: Total Image Programs Series (*TIPS*) and now, A New Weigh in 21 Days!

# A New Weigh in 21 Days!

## -- About the Book --

Would you participate in an experience that can transform (change) your life, weight and image in 21 days?  Then you are ready for *A New Weigh in 21 Days!*  Yes, that's right, you will experience a new weight when you get over the emotional weight, the mental weight and, finally, the physical weight related to pounds.  This is it, the book that is designed to use proven methods, concepts and terms that, when practiced for just 21 days, can transform your weight permanently.  Get ready for a new weight and a new you.

This incredible book offers you a life of freedom, for it can be used not only to support and guide you in the experience of a new weight, but the concepts can be practiced and will change *any lifestyle* that creates blocks and/or barriers to your personal success.  You *can* get "over weight" for now and always.  Read the book, *stay the course, experience a New Weigh in 21 Days!*